D0710560

The Terry Lectures

. .

MEDICINE AND HUMAN WELFARE

MEDICINE
AND
HUMAN WELFARE

BY

HENRY E. SIGERIST, M.D., D.Litt.

WILLIAM H. WELCH PROFESSOR OF HISTORY OF
MEDICINE IN THE JOHNS HOPKINS UNIVERSITY

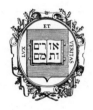

NEW HAVEN · YALE UNIVERSITY PRESS

LONDON · HUMPHREY MILFORD · OXFORD UNIVERSITY PRESS

1941

THE
DWIGHT HARRINGTON TERRY
FOUNDATION

LECTURES ON RELIGION IN THE LIGHT
OF SCIENCE AND PHILOSOPHY

THIS volume is based upon the sixteenth series of lectures delivered at Yale University on the Foundation established by the late Dwight H. Terry of Plymouth, Connecticut, through his gift of $100,000 as an endowment fund for the delivery and subsequent publication of "Lectures on Religion in the Light of Science and Philosophy."

The deed of gift declares that "the object of this Foundation is not the promotion of scientific investigation and discovery, but rather the assimilation and interpretation of that which has been or shall be hereafter discovered, and its application to human welfare, especially by the building of the truths of science and philosophy into the structure of a broadened and purified religion. The founder believes that such a religion will greatly stimulate intelligent effort for the improvement of human conditions and the advancement of the race in strength and excellence of character. To this end it is desired that lectures or a series of lectures be given by men eminent in their respective departments, on ethics, the history of civilization and religion, biblical research, all sciences and branches of knowledge which have an important bearing on the subject, all the great laws of nature, especially of evolution . . . also such interpretations of literature and sociology as are in accord with the spirit of this Foundation, to the end that the Christian spirit may be nurtured in the fullest light of the world's knowledge and that mankind may be helped to attain its highest possible welfare and happiness upon this earth . . .

"The lecturers shall be subject to no philosophical or religious test and no one who is an earnest seeker after truth shall be excluded because his views seem radical or destructive of existing beliefs. The founder realizes that the liberalism of one generation is often conservatism in the next, and that many an apostle of true liberty has suffered martyrdom at the hands of the orthodox. He therefore lays special emphasis on complete freedom of utterance, and would welcome expressions of conviction from sincere thinkers of differing standpoints even when these may run counter to the generally accepted views of the day. The founder stipulates only that the managers of the fund shall be satisfied that the lecturers are well qualified for their work and are in harmony with the cardinal principles of the Foundation, which are loyalty to the truth, lead where it will, and devotion to human welfare."

PREFACE

LIKE other Terry Lecturers I had to overcome considerable hesitation before I could accept the invitation to deliver a series of "Lectures on Religion in the Light of Science and Philosophy," being neither a theologian, nor a philosopher, nor even a religious man, at least not in the conventional sense of the word.

The deed of gift of the Dwight Harrington Terry Foundation, however, is conceived so broadly and in such a liberal spirit as to permit of any honest endeavor that is concerned with the improvement of human conditions. There can be no doubt that health and disease are factors that determine human welfare to a very large extent, and at all times the physician by fighting disease and promoting health has contributed powerfully to bettering the conditions of the individual as well as of society at large. Health is not a goal in itself, but disease is a shackle that has often prevented man from accomplishing his task on earth and from attaining his goal. The world has been deprived of endless spiritual values by the illness and premature death of creative individuals. In providing conditions for physical and mental health the physician, therefore, is contributing not only to the material welfare of society but also to its cultural development.

Medicine today is in a period of transition. During the last hundred years medical science has progressed more than ever before in history. It has forged new and powerful weapons for the conquest of disease, but we have not yet learned how to use them in a society whose structure has changed basically in the past century. In spite of all progress we still carry a heavy burden of unnecessary sickness, and large sections of our population have no, or certainly not enough, medical care.

There is a great deal of unrest in the medical world as a result of this paradoxical situation. While some physicians are fully aware of the trends of the time and have the courage to face the problem openly and to seek its best possible solution, others are afraid of any change. They look back to a past that is gone irrevocably. Trained as highly specialized and efficient scientists, they are unprepared to grapple with problems that are primarily social and economic. They have built for themselves a legendary, sentimental, and romantic history of their profession to which they cling desperately and which determines their actions.

The purpose of this little book is to discuss the manifold relations between medicine and human welfare and to clarify the present situation of public health by analyzing it historically and sociologically. Every situation is the result of definite historical developments, and unless we are aware of them we cannot understand the world in which we live, nor can we play our part intelligently.

The historian's work is comparable to that of the psychiatrist. The psychiatrist, by analyzing a patient, often endeavors to make him aware of unconscious patterns of behavior so that he may face them openly and thus get rid of them. In the same way the historian, by analyzing historical developments, often tries to reveal and clarify unconscious social trends, so that by facing and discussing them openly we may improve conditions through intelligent action.

The historian of medicine wants to know what has happened in the past and what is happening today. He endeavors to understand the phenomena of health and disease and their significance for the individual and society. In doing this, in not merely accepting the facts as they present themselves but in reflecting about them and trying to interpret them, he imperceptibly enters the field of philosophy.

Throughout its history medicine always had very close relationships with religion, as will become evident from the following discussion. And even in our day, when medicine has become a matter of science, is not the attempt to promote human welfare, to help in building a better world not in heaven but on earth, an effort that is not so very far from religion, although it excludes the transcendental?

All this may justify the presentation of these lectures under the auspices of the Terry Foundation.

HENRY E. SIGERIST

The Johns Hopkins University,
  November, 1940.

CONTENTS

ILLUSTRATIONS

MEDICINE AND HUMAN WELFARE

I. DISEASE

MEDICINE and religion have one common origin. Man found himself surrounded by a hostile nature and threatened daily by mysterious forces. A storm broke out, a drought fell over the land, destroying the crops and leading to starvation and death. Or an epidemic swept over the region and people died by the thousands. The life of primitive man was by no means happy and healthy, as some eighteenth-century philosophers believed. It was a ruthless, perpetual struggle between a brutal nature and as yet helpless mankind.

But man reacted against these forces that brought starvation, sickness, and death and were responsible for a great many of the unpleasant occurrences of everyday life. He believed them to be evil spirits, demons whose very function it was to cause harm, or the souls of the dead seeking a way to return to earthly life. He protected himself by endeavoring to placate the spirits, to ward them off, and religion and magic were the means of achieving this.

Medicine is but one aspect of the age-old struggle between man and nature, and primitive medicine was by necessity religious and magical in character. As disease was caused by spiritual powers it was to be fought by spiritual means. The views about the origin of disease determined the physician's actions. The purpose of diagnosis was to ascertain who was responsible for the patient's illness, whether it was a man who had bewitched him or a demon that had taken possession of him. Prognosis meant to determine the intentions of the god in regard to a patient. The interpretation of *omina*, of signs, spontaneous or provoked, became a highly differentiated science that played an important part throughout antiquity. It was the more important because correct interpretation of omina permitted the experienced observer to counteract the evil sign and to exploit the lucky one. The purpose of therapy was to remove the cause of disease, to drive out a demon from a patient's body, or to remove the effect of magic by magical means. The physician of primitive society, the shaman, was priest and sorcerer in one.

Minor ailments required no explanation. They were the obvious result of overfeeding, exposure to heat or cold, or everyday injuries. They were treated by the patient himself or by his relatives with empirical means, with home remedies. This treatment was not considered medicine. It was the obvious course to take, just as a man eats when he is hungry and drinks when he is thirsty.

The most complete system of religious medicine is to be found in Babylonia and Assyria. All Babylonian science was closely linked to theology and its sole purpose was to teach what man had to do in order to keep the gods benevolent or to appease them had they been provoked. To achieve this the sorcerer-priest had to know the intentions of the gods and this was done by observing and interpreting omina. There was but one origin of disease: the gods who, either directly as a punishment for sin, or by means of evil spirits, inflicted it upon man. All the elements of primitive medicine are found again in Babylonia but on a tremendous scale and expressed in a great literature. Many evil spirits have names and individual characters such as Labartu, one of the chief demons; Asakku, who causes fevers; Ti'u, who brings headaches; Nirgal and Namtar, the spirits of plague; and many others. Their evil doings are pictured in many texts of great poetic value:

Cold and rain that minish all things,
They are the evil Spirits in the creation of Anu spawned.
Plague Gods, the beloved sons of Bel,
The offspring of Ninkigal.
Rending in pieces on high,
Bringing destruction below,
They are the Children of the Underworld.
Loudly roaring on high,
Gibbering below,
They are the bitter venom of the gods.
The great storms directed from heaven—those are they,
The owl, that hoots over a city—that is they,
They are the children born of Earth,
That in the creation of Anu were spawned.
The highest walls, the thickest walls,
Like a flood they pass.
From house to house they break through,
No door can shut them out,
No bolt can turn them back,
Through the door like a snake they glide,
Through the hinge like the wind they blow;
Estranging the wife from the embrace of a husband,
Snatching the child from the loins of a man,
Sending the man forth from his home.

They are the burning pain
That bindeth itself upon the back of a man.[1]

or the following:

> Seven are they, seven are they,
> In the Ocean Deep seven are they,
> Battening in Heaven seven are they,
> In the Ocean Deep as their home they were reared,
> Nor male or female are they,
> They are as the roaming windblast,
> No wife have they, no son do they beget;
> Knowing neither mercy nor pity,
> They hearken not unto prayer or supplication.
> They are as horses reared among the hills;
> The Evil Ones of Ea,
> Throne-bearers to the gods are they.
> They stand in the highway to befoul the path,
> Evil are they, evil are they!
> Seven are they, seven are they,
> Twice seven are they!
> By Heaven be ye exorcised! By Earth be ye exorcised![2]

Since the "cause" of disease was known there was no need for diagnosis, but then, as ever, the patient was deeply interested in a prognosis. He wanted to know what the gods had in store for him. And this was discovered by the observation and interpretation of omina such as were seen in the liver of sacrificed animals, the flickering of a flame, the motion of a drop of oil on water, or in dreams, or in the stars, or in abnormal births. Omina, however, were more than this;

1. R. Campbell Thompson, *The Devils and Evil Spirits of Babylonia* (London, 1903), I, 51–53.
2. *Ibid.*, pp. 77–79.

they were manifested also by the gods in what we call
the symptoms of disease, all those changes that the
priest-physician observed in the sick man. They too
called for interpretation and indicated whether illness
was going to be long or short, fatal or harmless. And
since omina had not only indicative but also causal
virtues they gave a lead for the treatment of disease.
This implicit inclusion of bodily symptoms among the
omina made it possible for the Babylonian physician
to gather a vast amount of sound clinical observations without ever abandoning the field of religious
medicine.

Given an exclusively spiritual cause of disease,
treatment that aimed at removing the cause was spiritual also. The magic power of the word, incantation
and exorcism, was its highest expression. Texts are numerous. Some, like the following, are simple prayers:

O mighty lord, hero, first-born of Nunamnir!
Prince of the Anunnaki, lord of the battle!
Offspring of Kutusar the mighty queen!
O Nirgal, strong one of the gods, the darling of Ninminna!
Thou treadest in the bright heavens, lofty is thy place!
Thou art exalted in the Underworld.
With Ea among the multitude of the gods inscribe thy
    counsel!
With Sin in the heavens thou seekest all things!
And Bil thy father has granted thee that the black-headed
    race, all living creatures,
The cattle of Nirgal, created things, thy hand should rule!
I ——, the son of ——, am thy servant!
The wrath of god and goddess are laid upon me!
Uprooting and destruction are in my house!
Since thou art beneficent, I have turned to thy divinity!

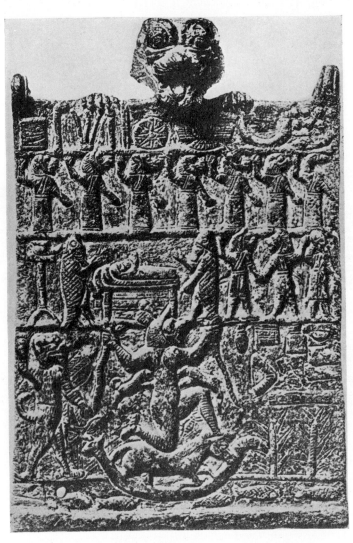

Fig. 1.

Treating a Patient through Incantation.

Assyrian relief.

Since thou art compassionate, I have sought for thee!
Since thou art pitiful, I have beheld thee!
Since thou art merciful, I have taken my stand before thee!
Truly pity me and hearken to my cries!
May thine angry heart have rest!
Loosen my sin, my offence
O god and angry goddess
Let me talk of thy greatness, let me bow in humility before
 thee![3]

Other texts give a graphic picture of the whole ritual
followed in such exorcism:

The Sorcerer-priest that maketh clear the ordinances of
 Eridu am I,
The Herald that goeth before Ea am I,
Of Marduk, sage magician and eldest son of Ea,
The Herald am I,
The Exorciser of Eridu, most cunning in magic am I;
O thou evil demon, turn thee to get hence,
O thou that dwelleth in ruins, get thee to thy ruins,
For the great lord Ea hath sent me;
He hath prepared his spell for my mouth
With a censer for those Seven, for clear decision,
He hath filled my hand.
A raven, the bird that helpeth the gods,
In my right hand I hold;
A hawk, to flutter in thine evil face,
In my left hand I thrust forward;
With the sombre garb of awe I clothe thee,
In sombre dress I robe thee
A glorious dress for a pure body.
O evil spirit, get thee hence,
Depart, O evil Demon!

3. Leonard W. King, *Babylonian Magic and Sorcery* (London, 1896), p. 89. See also A. Ungnad, *Die Religion der Babylonier und Assyrer* (Jena, 1921), p. 223.

From the body of the man, the son of his god,
O evil Demon, depart!
In the Temple of Ea stand not, nor circle around;
In the precincts of the house stand not, nor circle around;
"In the house will I stand," say thou not,
"In the precincts will I stand," say thou not,
"In the neighbourhood will I stand," say thou not,
O evil Spirit, get thee forth to distant places,
O evil Demon, hie thee unto the ruins,
Where thou standest is forbidden ground,
A ruined, desolate house is thy home;
Be thou removed from before me! By Heaven be thou exor-
    cised!
By Earth be thou exorcised![4]

Animal, vegetable, and mineral drugs were not unknown to the Babylonians, and we have records of several hundreds of them. But even their application had
often the character of a ritual, and there is no doubt
that theology dominated medicine.

It dominated also in the medical views of the ancient
Persians and Jews who both were strongly under
Babylonian influence. The Avesta and the Bible reveal ideas very similar to those of the Babylonians.
But while the belief in evil spirits, omina, and incantations was generally accepted and legitimate in Per-
sia, it was considered sinful and was fought by the
Jews. Monotheism and a purified cult had no room
for demons and exorcisms. But medicine was still religious. God has revealed his law. Whoever follows it in
piety will be rewarded and whoever sins will be punished. Disease, all suffering, is punishment for sin, of

4. R. Campbell Thompson, *loc. cit.*, I, 133–139.

the individual, of his parents, or of his clan. Such was the pitiless logic of Judaism. The remedies were lawful life, piety, atonement, and prayer.

We do not know what the beginnings of Egyptian medicine were, but there can be no doubt that it had a very different character. It was far more sober, was more a craft than a religion. Of the medical papyri preserved, one—the Edwin Smith Papyrus—is purely surgical, the manual of a craftsman. The other great papyri, Ebers, Hearst, and Brugsch Maior, contain some prayers and incantations but they are by no means in the foreground. The chief content of the books is rational, consisting of the description of disease symptoms and prescriptions of drugs. To be sure, there was religious and magical medicine in Egypt also, and the Ebers Papyrus explicitly mentions the three types of healers: physician, Sachmet-priest, and exorcist.[5] The latest medical papyri that have come down to us, Brugsch Minor and the Berlin Papyrus, are frankly magical. Since our material is scanty it is hard to tell whether there was a development from rational to magical medicine or whether both ran side by side through the centuries.

Religious medicine was much more widespread in the late Roman period than in the early days of Greece, a fact which suggests that mysticism and superstition flourish whenever a civilization is becoming old. Herodotus, on the other hand, speaks of the large number of medical specialists that he found in Egypt,

---

5. *Papyrus Ebers* 99, 2–3. B. Ebbell interprets "Sachmet-priest" as "surgeon," which is possible.

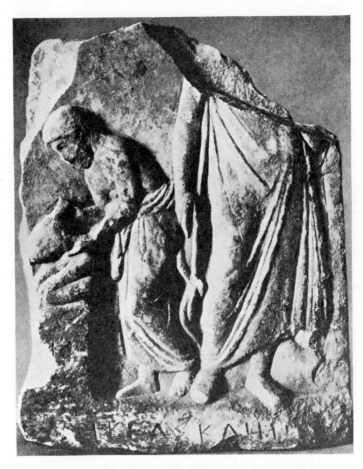

Fig. 2.

Miracle Cure in a Temple of Asklepios.

Votive relief from the Asklepieion in Athens.

specialists who certainly were neither priests nor sor-
cerers, and at that time Egyptian physicians were famous, their services being sought all over the ancient
world. I am therefore inclined to assume that it is due
to mere chance that the older manuscripts preserved
are rational and the younger magical and that both
forms of medicine actually existed side by side.

The Greeks developed a system of medicine that
excluded the transcendental and was based on observation and philosophic reasoning. With them medicine
was not only a craft but also a philosophic discipline,
part of the general learning; and nobody could claim
to be a scholar unless he had some knowledge of medicine. The Greeks made the two greatest discoveries in
medical history, namely, that disease is a natural
process, not basically different from physiological
processes, and further that the human body has an
innate healing power that endeavors to overcome lesions and to restore the lost balance of health. On the
basis of such views there grew up rational systems of
medicine that were closely connected with the various
philosophic schools.

But there was religious medicine in Greece also. It
centered for a long time in the cult of Asklepios, originally a local deity in northern Greece. When the Thes-
salians settled in the region they adopted the god and
spread his cult in the course of their migrations.

The legend of the healing god Asklepios was first
formulated by Hesiod around 700 B.C. Apollo one
day surprised Coronis—a virgin of the Lapithae—
bathing in Lake Boebeis. He conceived a passion for

her and possessed her. She became with child, but her father had chosen a husband for her, her cousin Ischys. What could she do but obey her father's will? The raven, Apollo's spy, brought news of the marriage. The wrathful god's first thought was to punish the bearer of evil tidings, and the bird which had hitherto been white bore thenceforward the hue of mourning. Ischys was slain by the arrows of Apollo, while the darts of Artemis laid Coronis and her innocent playmates low. Then, as Apollo contemplated the dead body of Coronis on the funeral pyre, he was struck with compassion for his unborn son, liberated the infant from the mother's womb, and took the babe to Mount Pelion, to the cave of Chiron the Centaur. There Asklepios grew to manhood, learning from his wise tutor which plants had healing virtues, and discovering many a charm that could cure illness. Thus he became a physician, greatly sought after. In the pride of his power, he ventured to transgress the laws of nature and to bring the dead back to life. Pluto, Lord of the Underworld, complained that Hades was being depopulated, and thereupon Zeus slew Asklepios with a thunderbolt.

In the legend the god treats patients by rational means such as herbs and the knife, and by μαλακαῖς ἐπαοιδαῖς, which can be translated in different ways. Wilamowitz[6] and others interpret it as charms or incantations while Edelstein[7] translates the words as

6. *Isyllos von Epidauros* (Berlin, 1886).
7. L. Edelstein, "Greek Medicine in Its Relation to Religion and Magic," *Bulletin of the Institute of the History of Medicine*, V (1937), 224 ff.

"kindly songs," which implies a treatment by music and makes Asklepios representative of a rational theology that stands in sharp opposition to a daimonic religion with magical rites. Indeed we know that music was applied in the treatment of diseases more than once in antiquity, particularly in the school of Pythagoras.

In the legend the god is destroyed for his presumption. The power he had over sick people induced him to overstep his limits and to resuscitate the dead. This expresses what the Greeks very strongly felt, namely, that it is not proper for the physician to interfere with the course of nature, that is a presumption only to be justified by necessity and imposes great responsibilities on the physician.

Conditions changed when the cult of Asklepios spread and became popular. The cures performed in Epidauros in the fourth century B.C. were miracle cures.[8] In the incubation the patient dreamed that he was treated by the god and found himself—sometimes —restored to health in the morning. It is possible, however, that in later centuries the priests of Asklepios combined dietetic treatments with religious rites.

Hippocratic medicine was rational, to be sure, but it had religious implications too.[9] What causes disease? Natural factors such as the sun, air, winds, or the nature of man, but these factors are conceived of as divine agencies. It is nature that cures the patient

8. R. Herzog, *Die Wunderheilungen von Epidauros* (Leipzig, 1931).

9. Edelstein, *loc. cit.*, p. 204 ff.

through its *vis medicatrix* and the physician is the helpmate of nature, which appeared to the Greeks as divine. When the physician makes a prognosis, when he foretells the patient's future, does he not assume the function of the prophet? Religious elements are mentioned, although rarely, in Hippocratic therapy. "Prayer indeed is good," says a Hippocratic writer, "but while calling on the gods a man should himself lend a hand."[10]

As time went on rational medicine became increasingly efficient. But religious medicine continued to develop. The cult of Asklepios spread and reached Rome in 293 B.C. Apollo entered the Roman world as the god of pestilence who when provoked sent plague by shooting his arrows at men, relieving them only when he had been placated. As Apello, the god who wards off disease, he was worshiped in the early days, and later his cult was introduced to the Gauls, where he was assimilated to local deities; for many centuries he remained plague god throughout the Roman Empire until Saint Sebastian took over his functions.[11]

One god after another assumed healing functions, and cures were performed in endless numbers of temples. Galen, the great physician of the second century A.D., himself sought healing in a temple of Asklepios. And noted hysterics like the rhetor Aristides spent years on pilgrimages from one temple to another.

10. M. P. E. Littré, *Œuvres complètes d'Hippocrate,* VI, 642.

11. See H. E. Sigerist, "Sebastian-Apollo," *Archiv für Geschichte der Medizin,* XIX (1927), 301–317.

In the ancient world, as everywhere, it was particularly those sick men whom scientific medicine had failed to cure who resorted to religion and magic. As Plutarch said: "Those who are ill with chronic diseases and do not succeed by the usual remedies and the customary diet turn to purifications and amulets and dreams."[12]

When Christianity came into the world it entered into competition with all the pagan healing cults, offering itself as the joyful gospel of the redeemer. The world was sick and in dire need of help. The new religion promised healing, both spiritual and physical restoration. Had not Christ himself performed cures? The language of the early literature of the church is full of references to medical matters.[13] The Christian writer Origen, refuting attacks on the new religion by the Roman philosopher Celsus, quite seriously discussed the question whether the true healer was Asklepios or Christ. His chief arguments in favor of Christ were that he had performed more cures, that his personality was closer to man, and that he had addressed himself to everybody, not only to the pure but also to the sinner. And this is the point. The ancient cults were for the healthy and sound. At the entrance of the sanctuary of Asklepios in Epidauros was the inscription:

> Pure must be he who enters the fragrant temple;
> Purity means to think nothing but holy thought.[14]

12. *De facie in orbe lunae,* 920b. Edelstein, *loc. cit.,* p. 244.
13. A. Harnack, *Medicinisches aus der ältesten Kirchengeschichte* (Leipzig, 1892).
14. Porphyrius, *De abstinentia animae,* II, 19.

The Christian religion, however, appealed to everybody and particularly to the disinherited, to the im-

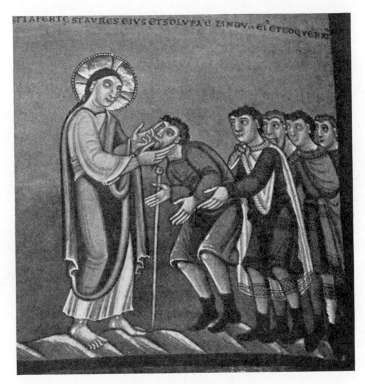

Fig. 3.

Christ Healing a Deaf-Mute.

From a manuscript of the Escorial.

pure, the sick and sinners, to the simple minded, to slaves and women. It promised them healing and redemption, an eternal life in glory. This was an attitude that shocked educated Romans deeply and Celsus declared that a bandit recruiting people for his gang could not make a better choice. But it was this attitude that gave Christianity its strong appeal at a time when many millions of people lived unattended and unaided in poverty, sickness, and oppression. And I think that this attitude is largely responsible for the fact that the new faith did not remain one of the many local Syrian sects but spread rapidly in the Roman Empire and became ultimately its official religion.

The significance of disease changed, and with it the position of the sick man in society. He was no longer burdened with the odium of sinfulness; disease no longer made him an inferior being, to be abandoned by his fellowman if the illness or disability could not be cured. It now gave him a preferential position in society. Through baptism a man became a member of a family, and just as the physical family recognized its responsibility toward the weak and poor member, so did the family of Christians. It was the Christian's duty to attend and nurse the sick fellow-Christian and to pray with him. The bishop as father of the family was in charge of charitable works. And when Christianity spread and became the official religion of the state, its family likewise grew to embrace society as a whole. From that time on the duty of society to care for the poor and for the sick was never disputed, even when it was not fulfilled.

Christian doctrine and Hellenistic science seemed irreconcilable. Christian medicine was faith healing.

Christ had "cured many of their infirmities and plagues and of evil spirits,"[15] and he had done it without the aid of drugs. There was no room for the physician in early Christian society, which believed that not study but the Spirit of God gave man the "gift of healing."[16] It was the prayer of faith that saved the sick, and the Lord raised him up. The elders of the church prayed over the ailing man, "anointing him with oil in the name of the Lord."[17] In the second century A.D. Christian students of Galen were excommunicated for devoting their time to the study of pagan medicine.[18]

A great deal of interpretation was required to justify the physician and to reconcile Christian faith with ancient medicine. This was done by quoting the words of Ecclesiastes: *"Honora medicum propter necessitatem, etenim illum creavit Altissimus. . . . Altissimus creavit de terra medicinam et vir prudens non abhorrebit illa."*[19]

Cassiodorus, the great chancellor of Theodoric, declared it meritorious for clerics to study and copy ancient books. His library in Vivarium contained works of Greek physicians in Latin translation. His views determined the cultural policies of the Benedictine order and it was largely due to him that the Greek tradition was not interrupted in the early Middle Ages. In the Benedictine abbeys sick people were nursed, but more than that, ancient medical books

15. Luke 7.21.   16. 1 Corinthians 12.9.
17. James 5.15, 14.
18. Eusebius, *Historia Ecclesiastica,* V, 28.
19. In the Vulgate, ch. xxxviii, 1, 4.

were copied, compilations and digests were made, and
the body of ancient science so far as it was available
in the Latin language was preserved and transmitted
to future generations. Christian charity and Greek
medicine combined and determined the course of the
healing art of the Middle Ages.

Greek rational therapy had an easy victory over
Christian faith healing, but medieval medicine never
lost the marks of its religious origin. Together with
the scientific precepts of Greek medicine it assimilated
the religious views and magical procedures of past
centuries and millennia. Epidemics were still ascribed
to the wrath of God and insanity to possession by
demons. Hellenistic incantations, charms, and amulets survived in Christianized form, while incubation
was practiced on Greek islands until the eighteenth
century.

In the Renaissance a strong trend toward realism
becomes noticeable. A new conception of science is
born which from the seventeenth century on develops
with increasing rapidity. Science gives man power
over nature and with every century more natural
forces are subjugated so as to serve man's purposes.
From then on the fight against disease is conducted
with scientific weapons and the doctor is no longer a
priest, nor even a mere craftsman, but a man of
science.

To our very day, however, religious medicine has
persisted. Today, as centuries ago, there are patients
who seek healing not with the doctors but in the
church. In every man's life there comes a disease

against which there is *nulla herba in ortis*. Where
science has reached its limits a miracle is hoped for.
In the Catholic Church religious medicine assumed
definite forms which are highly reminiscent of pagan
rites. Saints took on the healing functions of ancient
deities, and votive offerings representing organs or
diseased conditions were dedicated to them by grate-
ful patients as they had been in the temples of Asklepios.

Even in the Protestant Church healing cults sprang
up, such as Christian Science and New Thought.
They differ from the Catholic cults in that they do
not reflect pagan rites but are based consciously on
the faith healing of the early church. It is not by accident that Christian Science developed in America in
the late nineteenth and early twentieth centuries. It
was the time when American medicine became scientific and made the laboratory the temple of medicine.
This led to a neglect of psychological factors, and
Christian Science stepped into the gap. Modern psy-
chiatry, by stressing the psychological element of disease, has undermined the influence of these cults. They
still exist but hardly grow, and serve the needs of a
minority.

The fact that religious medicine has existed in all
periods of history shows that there must be definite
relations between the phenomena of illness and the
motives of religion, relations that must be examined.
Why is it that medicine was always so much closer to
religion than were other arts and crafts such as technology or agriculture?

To be sure, there have been religious and magical elements in technology also. A pot cracked in the oven, and to the primitive potter the most logical explanation was that the accident resulted from witchcraft. Alchemy, a mixture of chemistry, religion, and magic, owed its driving force to man's age-old yearning for eternal youth and wealth. The transmutation of one substance into another seemed a mystery. Like the physician, the alchemist, with his knowledge and skills, interfered with the regular processes of nature. Alchemy very often had much more the character of a religious movement than of a craft. Chemical operations became symbols; the attraction and repulsion of elements were given human values and considered as expressions of love and hatred. All alchemists were mystics—or charlatans. We also find that certain delicate technical processes, such as the casting of bells, were for a long time performed with definite rites.

With the advancement of science, however, technology lost its mystical elements. The engineer began to assume full control of all factors involved, and failures were explained scientifically.

The relations to religion are much closer in agriculture, where success or failure often depends on uncontrollable factors. Since the farmer is unable to control weather, for example, by scientific means, he may feel inclined to obtain power over it by religious or magical means—through prayer, sacrifices, or magic rites. Most primitive tribes have complicated dances to conjure rain, and church processions for rain can still be seen in backward farming popula-

tions. Agriculture, moreover, produces food which is
the source of life. The transformation of dead matter
into living substance able to nourish others and to re-
produce itself seemed a profound mystery. As a matter of fact, the process has not yet been explained scientifically, although there is no reason why we should
not be able to explain it some day. W. M. Stanley's
studies on the crystallization of viruses have opened
up new horizons and still further reduced the gap between organic and inorganic substances. But every
action of the farmer—ploughing, sowing, reaping,
harvesting—was performed for thousands of years
under sanction of religious and magical rites which
have survived to the present day, not only among
primitive tribes but also in old-stock peasant populations, rites that can be traced far back to pre-Chris-
tian days. And our eating and drinking customs still
bear the traces of early rituals.

Medicine, however, in its entire history was still
more intimately connected with religion. Why? Let
us first answer the question: what is disease? Disease,
as we have seen before, can be interpreted in very different ways. To us it is a biological process: our organism functions in response to stimuli which ema-
nate from the environment and from the organism
itself. These stimuli vary in their intensity, and the
organism is able to adapt itself to the changed conditions, as long as they do not exceed certain limits.
When we run, our muscles perform more work than
usual and therefore require more oxygen. We adapt
ourselves and answer the need by breathing more fre-

quently and by an increase in the number of heart-beats. The functions are still normal or physiological. When, however, stimuli exceed the adaptability of the organism, a lesion results and the reactions are no longer the normal ones but are morbid or pathological in character. The organism has available a set of reactions that tend to overcome lesions. Abnormal stimuli, however, and lesions may be or may become such that the organism is helpless, and in these cases the pathological reactions will be signs of degenerative processes. Disease is nothing else but the sum total of abnormal reactions of the organism or of its parts to abnormal stimuli.

Disease, then, is a biological process. Its phenomena therefore belong to the realm of science. But this process takes place in man, and thus always involves the mind. Sickness becomes an experience that affects man's welfare considerably. Disease, a destructive process that threatens life, may destroy only a few cells that can easily be replaced, but it may destroy the entire organism and with it the individual. For this reason, man suffers and is afraid: disease reminds him that he is mortal, that he must die sooner or later, and, if the illness is serious, it may be very soon. Disease interferes with the normal course of his life and brusquely interrupts the rhythm of his daily routine. The sick man is helpless; he cannot move as he is accustomed to do, cannot work, and becomes dependent on other people, his family or neighbors, or society at large. Civilization, which has placed at our disposal a variety of technical means for the control of nature,

seems helpless here. The sick man cannot avail himself
of these means. Disease, in other words, is a reversal
to primitivism and its victim is like a primitive man,
not only physically but often mentally also. Elementary fears, age-old views, come from the depth of the
unconscious, breaking through the thin crust of education. Rationalists become mystics, and it has happened more than once that sick physicians who knew
what was happening to them have become as supersti-
tious as an old peasant woman.

The helplessness of the sick man, the limitations of
medical science, and the proximity of death explain
the relationship between medicine and religion. They
explain why the natural process of disease has for
centuries been surrounded by a halo of mystery.

Since disease is an experience to the patient, the
artist who is the most sensitive of men and who recre-
ates his experiences in his works must of necessity re-
act strongly to illness.[20] There is a definite relationship
between an artist's illness and his creations, although
it is difficult to define. Mozart's productivity may be
partly explained by the fact that he suffered from tuberculosis. His life was to be short and little time was
given to him to express all the emotions that filled his
heart. And when the end was close he wrote his most
profound composition, the "Requiem."

The painter Watteau also suffered from tuberculosis for many years and died at the age of thirty-

20. H. E. Sigerist, "The Historical Aspect of Art and Medicine,"
Bulletin of the Institute of the History of Medicine, IV (1936),
286 ff.

seven. To me there is no doubt that his work, particularly his choice of subjects, was influenced by his illness. The many gallant ladies playing lightheartedly, the Italian comedians, the martial soldiers, are they not the expression of a man's pining for a life from which he was inexorably excluded, the outburst of a sick man who knew that his life was doomed?

The course of Van Gogh's mental illness can be traced in his paintings from his early creations to the "Black Birds." It was not his psychosis that made him an artist of genius, but disease and art were both expressions of the personality which, sick or normal, must reflect itself in his creations.

Mental patients who never had any special instruction frequently have the urge to express their feelings and thoughts in drawings, paintings, or sculptures. These creations provide an important clue to the understanding of their mental mechanisms and give access to their subconscious. Psychoanalysis is paying great attention to these artistic productions, and has developed their interpretation into a method of examination.[21] Many of these crude works of art remind us of the styles of definite historical periods, and an analysis of the mental processes responsible for such creations is of great interest not only to the physician but also to the student of art.

A serious illness is a great experience in the life of an individual, and in the same way a collective illness,

21. Hans Prinzhorn, *Bildnerei der Geisteskranken* (2d ed. Berlin, 1923). H. G. Baynes, *Mythology of the Soul, a Research into the Unconscious from Schizophrenic Dreams and Drawings* (Baltimore, 1940).

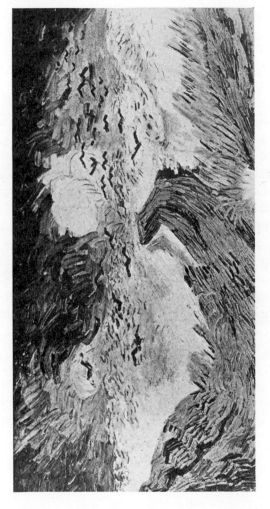

Fig. 4.

Van Gogh, The Black Birds.

an epidemic, is an experience in the life of a social group. The plague-ridden city has been described many times from Thucydides to Boccaccio and modern writers. And whether the pestilence was typhus or plague or yellow fever made little difference, the so-

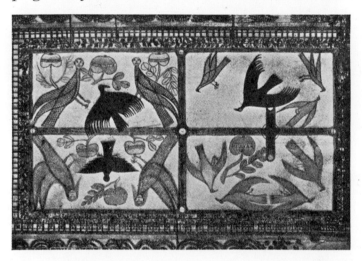

Fig. 5.

Painting by a Mental Patient.

(From Prinzhorn)

cial and psychological effects were very much the same. Nobody has described them more graphically than Boccaccio in the introduction to the *Decameron:*

Some thought that moderate living and the avoidance of all superfluity would preserve them from the epidemic. They formed small communities, living entirely separate from everybody else. They shut themselves up in houses where

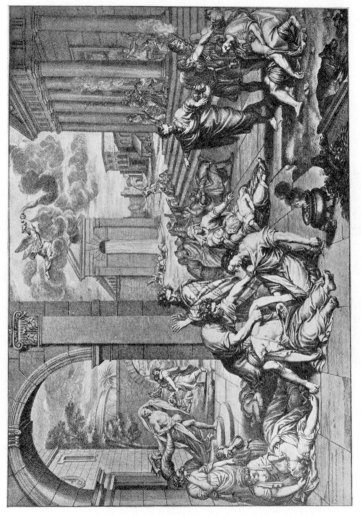

Fig. 6.

The Plague.

From an engraving of Mignard.

there were no sick, eating the finest food and drinking the best wine very temperately, avoiding all excess, allowing no news or discussion of death and sickness, and passing the time in music and suchlike pleasures. Others thought just the opposite. They thought the sure cure for the plague was to drink and be merry, to go about singing and amusing themselves, satisfying every appetite they could, laughing and jesting at what happened. They put their words into practice, spent day and night going from tavern to tavern, drinking immoderately, or went into other people's houses, doing only those things which pleased them. This they could easily do because everyone felt doomed and had abandoned his property, so that most houses became common property and any stranger who went in made use of them as if he had owned them. And with all this bestial behaviour, they avoided the sick as much as possible.

In this suffering and misery of our city, the authority of human and divine laws almost disappeared, for, like other men, the ministers and the executors of the laws were all dead or sick or shut up with their families, so that no duties were carried out. Every man was therefore able to do as he pleased.

Many others adopted a course of life midway between the two just described. They did not restrict their victuals so much as the former, nor allow themselves to be drunken and dissolute like the latter, but satisfied their appetites moderately. They did not shut themselves up, but went about, carrying flowers or scented herbs or perfumes in their hands, in the belief that it was an excellent thing to comfort the brain with such odours; for the whole air was infected with the smell of dead bodies, of sick persons and medicines.

Others again held a still more cruel opinion, which they thought would keep them safe. They said that the only medicine against the plague stricken was to go right away from them. Men and women, convinced of this and caring about nothing but themselves, abandoned their own city, their own houses, their dwellings, their relatives, their property, and went abroad or at least to the country round Florence, as if God's wrath in punishing men's wickedness with this plague would not follow them but strike only those who remained within the walls of the city, or as if they thought nobody in the city would remain alive and that its last hour had come.

When yellow fever ravaged the city of Philadelphia in 1793 scenes occurred that were reminiscent of those described by Boccaccio in Florence. A bookseller and publisher, Mathew Carey, gave a vivid account of them:

The consternation of the people of Philadelphia at this period was carried beyond all bounds. Dismay and affright were visible in almost every person's countenance. Most of those who could by any means make it convenient, fled from the city. Of those who remained, many shut themselves up in their houses, and were afraid to walk the streets. The smoke of tobacco being regarded as a preventative, many persons, even women and small boys, had segars almost constantly in their mouths. Others placing full confidence in garlic, chewed it almost the whole day; some kept it in their pockets and shoes. Many were afraid to allow the barbers or hair-dressers to come near them, as instances had occurred of some of them having shaved the dead—and many having engaged as bleeders. Some, who carried their caution pretty far, bought lancets for themselves, not daring to be bled with the lancets of the bleeders. Many houses were hardly a moment in the day free from the smell of gunpowder, burned tobacco, nitre, sprinkled vinegar, &c. Some of the churches were almost deserted, and others wholly closed. The coffee house was shut up, as was the city library, and most of the public offices—three out of the four daily papers were discontinued, as were some of the others. Many were almost incessantly employed in purifying, scouring, and whitewashing their rooms. Those who ventured abroad, had handkerchiefs or sponges impregnated with vinegar or camphor at their noses, or smelling-bottles full of the thieves' vinegar. Others carried pieces of tarred rope in their hands or pockets, or camphor bags tied round their necks. The corpses of the most respectable citizens, even of those who did not die of the epidemic, were carried to the grave, on the shafts of a chair, the horse driven by a negro, unattended by a friend or relation, and without any sort of ceremony. People hastily shifted their course at the sight of a hearse coming towards them. Many never walked on the foot path, but went into the middle of the streets, to avoid being infected in passing by houses wherein people had died. Acquaintances and friends avoided each other in the streets, and only signified their regard by a cold nod. The old custom of shaking hands fell into such general disuse, that many shrunk back with affright at even the offer of the hand. A person with a crape, or any appearance of mourning, was shunned like a viper. And many valued themselves highly on the skill and address with which they got to windward of every person whom they met. Indeed it is not probable that London, at the last stage of the plague, exhibited stronger marks of terror, than were to be seen in Philadelphia, from the 25th or 26th of August, till pretty late in September. When people summoned up resolution to walk abroad, and take the air, the sick cart conveying patients to the hospital, or the hearse carrying the dead to the grave, which were travelling almost the whole day, soon damped their spirits, and plunged them again into despondency.[22]

Similar scenes can be observed in our own times. I remember a day in the summer of 1918 when the epidemic of influenza was at its height. I was in the Swiss

22. *A Short Account of the Malignant Fever Lately Prevalent in Philadelphia* . . . (4th ed. Philadelphia, 1794), p. 214.

Army Medical Corps and had to report at headquar-
ters. When I came to the small city of Porrentruy I
found myself all of a sudden in a medieval atmosphere
of terror and panic. The first sight was a huge stack
of new coffins at the railroad station. In the city the
population was in a state of tension and extreme
nervousness. Many were weeping in the streets. Some
had relatives dying at home, others feared for their
own lives. The wildest rumors were circulating and
found all-too-credulous ears. Alcoholic drinks were
supposed to protect against the disease and people
were seen drunk in the streets in the early morning.
According to another rumor the workers of the local
tobacco factory had been spared and I saw women
with huge cigars who had never smoked before. Whenever a person was buried the church bells were rung,
and this permanent ringing of bells added to the terror of the population. Physicians were scarce; they
were sick themselves or in the army, and since I was
in the uniform of an army physician I was dragged
into dozens of houses and was almost kidnaped, so
that I could hardly fulfil my task. People clung to the
physicians and expected miracles from them, not re-
alizing how helpless we were. A few months later, on
an epidemiological survey I came to an Alpine hut,
high up in the mountains, and found all the inhabitants dead. It was a horrible sight, the bodies livid
and in the early stages of decomposition. Terrified,
my guides muttered, "The Black Death"—which it
was clinically if not etiologically.

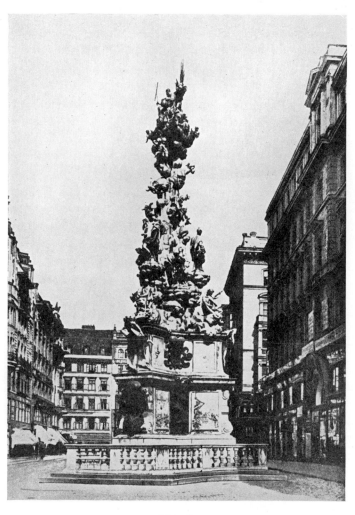

Fig. 7.

Plague Column in Vienna.

In other words, when a pestilence, whatever it may be, strikes a people, the reaction is virtually the same today as it was in former centuries.

The anxiety and sufferings endured by a community during a visitation of the plague are responsible for the creation of many works of art. Altars and churches such as Santa Maria della Salute, in Venice, were vowed when a plague was at its height and erected when the epidemic had died out.

The Greek world exalted the healthy and sound and considered disease the sign of an inferior being. In the Christian world there was a definite tendency to glorify suffering and to look up to the sick and suffering man as to a superior being. Christ crucified, through his agony and death, had redeemed the world. Whoever suffered was carrying the Cross in the footsteps of his Master. Suffering was interpreted as an ordeal and whoever stood the test without rebellion could expect to be rewarded in the hereafter. The story of the righteous Job suffering unrighteously, rebelling but then humbling himself and submitting to God, acquired increased significance. In Christianity *Pathos* became *Ethos*. Suffering was a sign of grace, not to be evaded but sought. People escaped the world, became ascetics, perched on columns, inflicted pain and mutilations on themselves.

This Christian interpretation of suffering was a comfort to the patient. The leper who was expelled from human society could be reconciled with his fate by being told that his would be a meritorious life for which he would be rewarded. Such an interpretation also answered the great question, Why? Why should an innocent man be sick and suffer? The Jewish explanation that it was in atonement for the sin of others could not satisfy a society that was familiar with the concepts of Roman law. Suffering, however, could be understood and borne with patience and humility as soon as it was looked upon as a trial sent by God for the benefit of the sufferer.

It was the Christian's duty not to inflict pain but to alleviate it whenever he found it. However, when suffering was glorified there was little incentive to fight it. If hell on earth meant paradise in heaven, why should conditions be changed? The Christian church preached love, but in almost two thousand years it failed to remove some of the basic causes of physical and mental suffering, of poverty, exploitation, social inequality, and injustice. A spiritual power in its origin, the church in the fourth century had allied itself with the temporal powers and thus lost its spiritual autonomy. It became the largest property owner and a temporal power itself. In more than one conflict it sided with the strong against the weak. It sent missionaries to Africa to convert the negroes and blessed the white man who exploited them.

In medieval literature the sick man is sometimes pictured as the normal man, in contrast with the healthy and sturdy individual, who appears as abnormal or certainly as inferior. Much later, in the romantic school, the frail tubercular woman and the chlorotic young girl were popular figures. Samuel Butler's *Erewhon*, the Utopian world in which illness is a criminal offense, punishable by law, was a wholesome reaction to this tendency.

Suffering is not in itself meritorious. It is an obvious indictment of society that we have not yet learned to apply science and social planning to the problem of unnecessary suffering. In a world that is ruled by iron economic necessity, unemployment is responsible for a vast amount of economic and moral distress. In countries where there is no sickness insurance protracted illness may degrade a man by making him a recipient of charity. If he recovers he may resume his old place in society, but if his illness has left the slightest disability his standard of living will drop. The skilled worker will join the ranks of the unskilled, or he may become permanently unemployable. Thus, disease creates poverty and poverty disease. The vicious circle is closed. One way to break it is by fighting disease with every scientific means available to us. It is better to do this now than to wait passively for social and economic adjustments which may overcome poverty and guarantee every family sufficient food and a decent home.

There is an iron rule which is valid everywhere, namely, that no individual and no family can lead a healthy and decent life unless they have a certain minimum income. If this is not provided by wages, somebody has to make up the balance. It may be the community that responds by providing social services such as housing, free distribution of milk to children, relief money, and similar services. If this is not done, people will of necessity become antisocial, may de-

velop illness or break the law, and in such cases society must pay a far greater bill by erecting and
operating hospitals and jails.

Illness, which cannot be foreseen but may strike a
family overnight, remains a permanent threat to human welfare and security, a threat that will only be
met more adequately when society devises some form
of insurance accessible to all.

Since many diseases are communicable, patients
suffering from them become a direct menace to their
neighbors. In such cases society, represented by the
state, feels justified in interfering with the individual
in order to protect itself. So we find that for many
centuries patients suffering from certain contagious
diseases have had to be reported to the authorities.

The European development of this trend began in
the early Middle Ages, when leprosy had become a serious social problem. Since physicians had no remedy
and were totally helpless, the church undertook to
protect society by applying principles described in
Leviticus. Greek medicine never had a clear understanding of contagion, but in Greece and throughout
the ancient world the spiritual condition of uncleanliness was considered contagious. The concept was de-
fined especially clearly in Leviticus but was by no
means restricted to the religion of Israel. According
to Leviticus an individual becomes unclean through
physiological processes such as menstruation and
childbirth or through pathological processes such as
discharge from the urethra. And this uncleanliness is
contagious. Whoever touches an unclean person, ani-

mal, or object becomes unclean also and must undergo
definite purification rites. Nobody was compelled to
be pure but the unclean individual was isolated socially, as a source of uncleanliness to others, and was
excluded from the temple. Unclean to a particularly
severe degree were people suffering from çara'ath, a
disease condition which in all probability included our
leprosy. Such patients had to be reported to the
priests, were examined, and in dubious cases isolated
temporarily and reëxamined. If their condition was
established beyond any doubt, they were segregated,
and thenceforth excluded from human society. "And
the leper in whom the plague is, his clothes shall be
rent, and his head bare, and he shall put a covering
upon his upper lip, and shall cry: Unclean, unclean.
All the days wherein the plague shall be in him he
shall be defiled; he is unclean: he shall dwell alone;
without the camp shall his habitation be."[23]

In the Middle Ages the church organized the fight
against leprosy by following these precepts and in so
doing it stamped the lepers as patients of a special
kind. The leper was a man who on account of his illness was considered a threat to his fellowmen and was
declared unfit for normal social life. He was segregated—and still is in many countries—and lost his
civic rights. Since his illness was incurable he was an
outcast for life and was dead socially long before
physical death had released him.

It was observed in the Middle Ages that there were
other diseases which were spread through contagion.

23. Leviticus 13.45–46.

Bernard of Gordon in the early fourteenth century
lists them in two verses of his *Lilium Medicinae:*

> *Febris acuta, ptisis, scabies, pedicon, sacer ignis,*
> *Anthrax, lippa, lepra nobis contagia praestant.*[24]

When the Black Death invaded the Western World
it was combated on the same principles as leprosy.
Patients had to be reported to the authorities, were
examined, and isolated in their houses for the dura-
tion of their illness. If they died their personal effects
were burned or washed thoroughly with soap and exposed to the sun. Quarantines were established for the
temporary segregation of persons coming from infected areas. Like the leper, the plague-ridden man
was a patient of a special kind and was considered the
immediate concern of society. These same principles
were gradually extended to other epidemic diseases
and as more was learned about their cause and nature
the regulations became stricter. Today in all civilized
countries many diseases are reportable by law. Houses
in which such patients live are marked as a warning
to others, and patients suffering from such diseases
become the object of legislation. There are no laws
concerning gout or ulcers of the stomach, but whenever society feels itself menaced protection is sought
by all means available, and the interest of the individual must give way to the common welfare.

Vaccination laws testify to a still greater interfer-

24. The diseases are: acute fever diseases such as plague, tuberculosis, scabies, epilepsy, which for a long time was considered contagious, erysipelas, anthrax, ophthalmic gonorrhea or trachoma,
possibly both, leprosy.

ence with the individual sphere. It is undoubtedly a tremendous encroachment upon personal liberty to force the consent of an individual to being made sick artificially in order to protect him and his fellowmen from more serious illness. Vaccination with cowpox was described by Edward Jenner in 1798, and the development of vaccination laws coincided with a period of political liberalism which explains the enormous difficulties encountered in many countries in passing such legislation. There are still areas, such as Austria until very recently and most states of the United States,[25] where vaccination cannot be openly required, and must be sought by indirect methods. Vaccination is not compulsory but elementary education is and the schools do not admit children who are not vaccinated. The same difficulties are encountered in enforcing immunization against diphtheria, typhoid, and other diseases, and yet the advantage to the individual and to the community is obvious. The attitude of a society toward protective immunization is an excellent test of its health consciousness and sense of responsibility. It reveals how far a group has moved in the development from a competitive to a coöperative society.

A patient of a still more special kind is the one suffering from venereal diseases in those countries that have passed legislation to combat these diseases. As early as 1788 Denmark made the treatment of vene-

25. J. W. Kerr, "Vaccination, an Analysis of the Laws and Regulations Relating Thereto in Force in the United States," *Public Health Bulletin,* No. 52 (Washington, 1912).

real diseases compulsory and provided free medical
services to such patients, with the result that venereal
diseases, particularly syphilis, have practically disappeared. In 1927 Germany passed a very strict law.
Venereal diseases must be reported to the public
health authorities. Treatment is free but compulsory.
If a patient changes his residence while he is under
treatment, his moves are reported to the authorities
of his new domicile and he must continue treatment
there. Whoever knowingly contaminates another person may be punished by as much as three years' imprisonment. The result of this legislation was very
soon felt in a sharp decline in the incidence of venereal
diseases. The Soviet Union has passed similar laws
with equally good results. It is obvious, however, that
legislation alone has no effect unless it is combined
with education and the provision of all facilities required for prevention and cure.

The venereal patient, in other words, not only is in
the position of other contagious sick persons but he
also becomes a criminal offender if he knowingly
spreads his disease. This is a totally new attitude
which has developed only recently. The power of the
state is called upon to protect society against certain
diseases and to enforce health by very drastic means.
The professional secrecy that safeguards the privacy
of the patient is disregarded in such cases. There is a
marked tendency today to restrict the physician's ob-
ligation to secrecy; more than that, to impose upon
him the duty of divulging secrets if the welfare of
third persons or of society at large is involved. This

attitude is expressed unmistakably in the penal codes
of a number of countries.

In a coöperative society general welfare comes before individual welfare, and the more specialized society becomes the more we are obliged to give up certain individual liberties and to assume responsibilities
toward the social group of which we are a part. We
must pay taxes and must send our children to school,
whether we like it or not. If we build a house we must
conform with the city regulations. These are self-
imposed duties that we accept. But we must and shall
go further and learn to accept obligations in matters
of health and disease also. The soldier is not allowed
to mutilate himself or to acquire diseases that can be
prevented, and in the same way the citizen conscious
of his duties will accept measures that protect his and
his fellows' health.

We have seen that an epidemic is an acute social
illness. An entire group falls sick; some members of it
may succumb, the others recover, and after awhile the
epidemic is gone and usually forgotten. Measles break
out. The school children get it, carry it home, and in-
fect their brothers and sisters. A number of years
elapse until a new group of children with no immu-
nity reaches school age and the soil is ready for a new
outbreak of measles. There is also influenza, which
can be traced back to the thirteenth century. Once in
a generation, every thirty to forty years, the disease
fell upon mankind, killing off millions. There was a
time when it was attributed to the influence of the
stars, hence the name: *influentia astrorum*. It is al-

most safe to predict that we may expect a new pandemic outbreak of influenza between 1950 and 1960 when a generation will have grown up that was not affected by the epidemic of 1918–19.

But there are epidemic diseases that are not acute, that do not come and go, but reside permanently in a definite region. These are endemic diseases. Their agents are firmly entrenched in that region, living and developing at the expense of the inhabitants. Where such a disease prevails, the welfare and general standard of an entire population are most deeply affected. For more than two thousand years the history of the Roman Campagna has been determined by the presence or absence of malaria.[26] When the disease was at its height, life died out and when—for reasons unknown to us—the disease receded, the Campagna again became a flourishing landscape, teeming with life. The population of a malaria region is handicapped in all its activities. Quite apart from the menace to life, chronic malaria saps the vitality of the people, undermines their energies, breaks their initiative. The same is true of the hookworm disease. A miserable worm can stultify and degrade an entire population. Where such an endemic disease prevails, the activities of the people are reduced; their standard of living falls, poverty results, and the consequence is still more disease, other diseases. Once more the vicious circle is closed, not for the individual alone but for the entire group.

26. A. Celli, *The History of Malaria in the Roman Campagna* (London, 1933).

Disease is not a new phenomenon. It must be almost as old as life itself. At all times there must have been stimuli that exceeded the adaptability of an organism. Disease, we may say, is nothing but life—life under abnormal conditions. Paleopathology, by examining fossil bones of animals, has been able to demonstrate that disease occurred long before the advent of man. What is even more important, it could be proved that it occurred at all times in the same basic forms that are being observed today. The examination of Egyptian mummies has shown that such diseases as tuberculosis and arteriosclerosis attacked man at an early period of history. Clubfoot, rickets, and a variety of other diseases are depicted unmistakably in ancient Egyptian works of art.

The incidence of illness, however, varies in different regions and has changed a great deal in the course of time. The tropics have diseases peculiar to them. Goiter is, or was until very recently, a disorder characteristic of Alpine regions. Great social upheavals, wars and revolutions, were invariably accompanied by outbreaks of severe epidemics. Indeed, war, famine, and pestilence were, and still are, a standing triad of evils. In the Franco-Prussian War more people died from diseases than from wounds. In the World War for the first time no major epidemics occurred as a result of the war, at least on the Western Front. On the Eastern Front typhus ravaged armies and civilian population. The epidemic of influenza which killed ten million people all over the world was not a result of the war, although the massing of people

probably increased the death toll. In Russia, after
the Revolution, as a result of blockade, civil war, and
foreign intervention, famine and epidemics devastated
the country in a measure that had not occurred since
the Middle Ages or the Thirty Years' War.

The human mind interfered with the natural course
of disease. Education, public health, medicine and,
above all, a rising standard of living altered conditions radically. Life is far less hazardous today than
it has been in the past. A person born in the eighteenth century had good chances of dying from gastro-
intestinal diseases in the first weeks of life or as soon
as warm weather set in. Many children were born and
many died: in the average family it was rare for more
than two to reach maturity. Whatever surplus of
population was produced was killed off in wars. The
population of Germany was constant for a thousand
years, from Charlemagne to 1800, and amounted to
about 20 million. Between 1800 and 1900 it increased
to 56 million. The infantile death rate, that is, the
number of children dying in the first year of life for
every 1,000 children born, is between 30 and 70 in
most civilized countries. It was ten times higher in the
eighteenth century.

If a child at that time survived its diarrheas it was
then exposed to the many acute infantile diseases—
measles, whooping cough, scarlet fever, diphtheria—
which used to be infinitely more frequent and deadly
than they are today. In New York, in the fifty years
from 1870 to 1920, measles decreased by 84 per cent,
diphtheria by 97 per cent, typhoid by 95 per cent.

Diphtheria, once a much dreaded disease, is now preventable and there is no justification for it to exist at all. It is up to the population to get rid of it altogether.

The child who survived the infantile diseases and grew up to adolescence had good chances of acquiring tuberculosis. Phthisis was very common and attacked all classes of society. In 1857 in the State of Massachusetts, 450 persons out of every 100,000 died of tuberculosis. From then on the death rate dropped constantly. It was down to 250 in 1890, 114 in 1920, and was 35.6 in 1938. A similar downward trend can be observed in other regions, and tuberculosis is receding even in countries where hardly any measures are applied to combat it. Tuberculosis today has become a social disease, bred in slums, a disease of the low-income groups, or unskilled workers' families. This is why in the United States negro families are much more affected than white families. In Paris[27] in 1923–26 the sixteenth district inhabited by well-to-do families had an average death rate of 130 while the twentieth, a working-class district, had a rate of 340. The difference was still more pronounced in 1926, when the death rate was 75 in the rich eighth district and 306 in the poor thirteenth district. This proportion of one to four also applies in the United States to the white and colored populations. In 1924 a group of 17 house blocks in Paris with 4,290 houses and a population of 185,000 had the appalling death rate

27. The figures from P. Pierreville, *L'Inégalité humaine devant la mort et la maladie* (Paris, 1936).

of 480. Tuberculosis, therefore, remains a serious problem for large groups of the population, although as a whole conditions have greatly improved.

In the eighteenth century man was constantly menaced by a variety of infectious diseases that have practically disappeared today. During that period in London alone 2,000 people died every year from smallpox in spite of the fact that inoculation was already reducing the death rate. It has been estimated that in Europe in the eighteenth century from $\frac{1}{14}$ to $\frac{1}{12}$ of all deaths were caused by smallpox.[28] Diseases carried by water and food, such as typhoid and dysentery, were extremely widespread and were responsible for endless cases of disability and death. They can be controlled today and an epidemic of typhoid is not only a catastrophe but also a scandal. Cholera swept over the Western World three times in major epidemics during the nineteenth century, once in the 1830's, in the 1840's, and again in the 1890's. The first time health authorities were helpless and the disease took its course, but in the '90's the bacillus was found and the mode of transmission established. New water supplies were constructed and more recently a vaccine has been prepared that protects against cholera. The disease is no longer a problem in the West.

In the 1700's large sections of Europe and North America were infected with malaria which was attributed to exhalations from swamps. Epidemics broke

28. P. Kübler, *Geschichte der Pocken und der Impfung* (Berlin, 1901), p. 101.

out regularly in the autumn. Thousands of people were sick and many died. There was a remedy for the fever, the cinchona bark that came into general use in the seventeenth century. But the disease could not be attacked at its root until Laveran found the parasite that causes it and Ross described its transmission to men through mosquitoes. Through the destruction of mosquitoes and larvae, and through the draining of swamps where insects breed, the incidence of the disease has been reduced considerably and it is today as much an economic as a medical problem. Yellow fever, a disease dreaded all over the American continent, was also found to be transmitted by mosquitoes and was combated in a similar way.

If in the eighteenth century a man succeeded in surviving infantile diarrheas and the many acute infectious diseases of childhood; if he was spared by tuberculosis, smallpox, and a dozen other contagious diseases and reached the age of fifty, then his chances of attaining old age were about the same as today. Those who talk about the old people in the good old days usually forget to ask how many brothers and sisters they had and at what age they died.

There is no doubt that the general life expectancy has increased considerably. A child born in fifteenth-century Europe had an average life expectancy of from twenty to twenty-five years, while it is over sixty today, and in New Zealand over sixty-six. This tremendous increase, however, is primarily due to the reduction of infantile mortality and to the control of acute diseases affecting chiefly the first decades of life.

Improvement in health conditions is also expressed by the general death rate, which is the number of people dying in a year for every 1,000 population. It was never under 50 in the eighteenth century and is between 8 and 15 in the countries of Western civilization today. It was 17.6 in the United States in 1900 and was reduced to 11.5 in 1936, which means that 750,000 human lives were saved that year which would have been lost in 1900.

All these figures show that great progress has indeed been achieved in health matters, that life is noticeably less dangerous, and that human welfare is much less affected by disease than it was before. But let us not forget that these great improvements have benefited less than one half of the world's population. More than one billion human beings in Africa and Asia alone have health conditions today that are as bad as the worst conditions the Western World ever experienced.

And even in the advanced countries, are conditions as good as they could be? Is not illness still a very serious problem? Let us examine only one country, the United States, which as a result of unique circumstances has succeeded in establishing a relatively high material standard of living in many sections and where health conditions are generally recognized as good.[29]

29. The following figures are taken from the *Report of the Technical Committee on Medical Care,* accepted and endorsed by the Interdepartmental Committee to Coördinate Health and Welfare Activities, presented to the President, February 14, 1938. (Washington, 1938.)

The decrease in the incidence of tuberculosis has already been mentioned. With 50.6 in 1936 the United States has one of the lowest death rates in the world. However, if we have human welfare in mind we must not think in terms of rates alone but must face the absolute figures as well. The low death rate still means that an average of 70,000 people die of tuberculosis annually, that about 420,000, almost half a million, suffer from it, and that one million other people are directly exposed to infection. There is no doubt, therefore, that the disease still presents a serious problem and is a great threat, particularly to the age group from fifteen to forty-five years.

The situation is worse in the case of venereal diseases where America is far behind European countries. Over a million people seek treatment annually for gonorrhea, over half a million for syphilis. More than 60,000 children are born with the handicap of congenital syphilis, while at least 10 per cent of all mental patients first admitted to hospitals are sick as a result of syphilitic infection. It is easy to realize how much physical and mental misery venereal diseases bring to individuals and to families.

Pneumonia disables over half a million people each year and kills about 150,000. New chemotherapeutic drugs have been prepared recently which promise to reduce the number of deaths from pneumonia quite considerably. But until now the problem has been serious and it is still far from solved.

Mental patients fill half a million, or one half of all hospital beds available in the country, and twice as

many outside of institutions show various degrees of
mental maladjustment.

The United States has a very low infantile death
rate. In the period 1934–36 it ranked seventh in the
world together with England and Wales. The first six
were New Zealand, Holland, Australia, Norway,
Switzerland, and Sweden. This low death rate, however, still means that nearly 70,000 infants die in the
first month of life, some 53,000 from the second to
the twelfth month, and if we add to this the 75,000
infants stillborn annually, it means that every year
198,000 young women go through the trying period
of pregnancy and childbirth and the result is a dead
child or one that will die very soon. And every year
14,000 women die from causes connected with pregnancy and childbirth, robbing families of the mother
and wife.

Since acute diseases attacking young people have
decreased so considerably, allowing more people to
reach maturity and old age, diseases peculiar to these
latter age groups have increased and chronic diseases
disabling people often for long periods of time are
much more frequent. Diseases of the heart, blood ves-
sels, and kidneys constitute the chief cause of death,
killing almost 600,000 people annually. The rate has
almost doubled since 1900. The same is true of can-
cer, from which about 400,000 people suffer, and
143,000 die annually.

But not only the deadly diseases affect human welfare. The numerous lesser ailments, the minor diseases
of the respiratory and digestive organs; the colds,

coughs, and sore throats; the stomach aches, diarrheas and constipations; the headaches and rheumatic pains; women's ailments and skin troubles, all of these disable millions of people. It has been estimated that in the United States on an average day four million people or over three per cent of the population are disabled by illness, and many more without interrupting their work are reduced in their efficiency and feel uncomfortable. The average person has from one to two disabling illnesses a year and loses about ten days from his work.

Illness, even in a country with good health conditions, not only causes endless suffering but is also a tremendous economic burden to the population. It has been estimated that the people of the United States lose not less than ten billion dollars every year on account of illness, including the cost of medical care, loss of earnings, and capital loss due to premature deaths.

II. HEALTH

AFTER having discussed disease and its significance for the welfare of the individual and society, we now approach the problems of health. We
feel tempted simply to reverse the picture drawn in
the preceding lecture and to declare that health is the
absence of disease and that its significance for human
welfare is the contrary of that of disease. Such a statement, however, would be utterly wrong because health
is immeasurably more than just the absence of disease. What then is it?

Most people are not aware of health and take it for
granted as long as they have it, becoming conscious
of it only when illness sets in, just as they are not
aware of having a stomach until they feel a pain in it.
Pain is an alarm signal which warns us that some part
of our body is threatened. Pain, a symptom of so
many diseases, compels us to realize that we were en-
joying health and that we are losing something that
now seems highly desirable. Absence of pain undoubtedly is an important factor of health but it is
only one factor. What then is health?

Many physicians tell us that it is impossible to give
an accurate definition of health. And yet they all
have, more or less consciously, a practical concept of
it. Otherwise they would be unable to treat patients.
They often have to determine whether a man is sick
or not and the immediate goal of their treatment is
the restoration of health. Therefore they must have

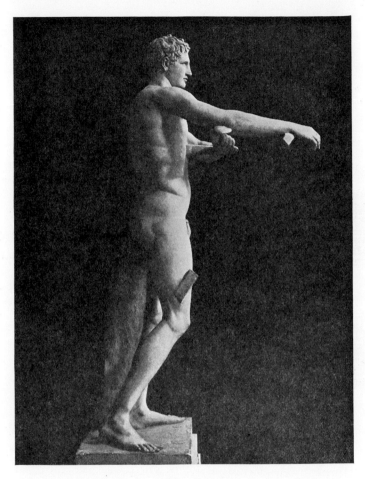

Fig. 8.

The Apoxyomenos of Lysippus.

Representing the Greek ideal of a harmonious body.

an idea of what it is, even if it is not formulated. It is
one weakness of our present system of medical education that health plays a very small part in it. The student's interest is directed primarily toward disease.[1]

In order to obtain a clear view of what health is
and what it means we must again attempt a historical
analysis. Our present concept is the result of a long
historical development. The attitude toward health
has changed a great deal in the course of time. While
it always seemed desirable to the individual, the degree of desirability and the motivations changed considerably. The valuation of health was determined by
the attitude toward the human body and by a variety
of religious and philosophic factors.

Again we must go back to the foundations of our
Western civilization, to ancient Greece. What seemed
most desirable to the Greek? In the early days the
Homeric hero prayed to the gods for glory, for a
long life, or possibly for a painless death.[2] But later,
in the sixth and still more in the fifth century B.C.,
the philosophers considered health one of the highest
goods. The testimonies are endless. "For mortal man
the highest good is to be healthy," was declared in an
old scolion.[3] In a dialogue ascribed to Plato[4] it is said
that it is better to have little money and to be healthy

1. See E. Stanley Ryerson, "Human Health and Its Assessi-
bility," *Journal of the Association of American Medical Colleges,*
XV (March, 1940), 91–97.
2. See Ludwig Edelstein's illuminating study "Antike Diätetik,"
Die Antike (1931), VII, 255–270, which I have used extensively in
discussing the ancient concept of health and ancient dietetics.
3. Attic Scolion 7, *Lyra Graeca,* III, 564. Loeb Classical Series.
4. Eryxias 393.

than to be sick with all the wealth of the great king;
and the poet Ariphron praised health in a paean:

Health, eldest of Gods, with thee may I dwell for the rest of
my life and find thee a gracious house-mate. If there be any
joy in wealth, or in children, or in that kingly rule that
maketh men like to Gods, or in the desires we hunt with the
secret nets of Aphrodite, or if there be any other delight or
diversion sent of Heaven unto man, 'tis with thy aid, blessed
Health, that they all do thrive and shine in the converse of
the Graces; and without thee no man alive is happy.[5]

This high valuation of health soon became general
and disease, therefore, was considered a curse, as we
have mentioned before. The Stoics endeavored to
overcome this view by declaring health and disease to
be *adiaphora*, indifferent matters. Virtue alone is a
good, wickedness alone an evil. But even the Stoics
had to make concessions to the general views, and in
its later development the school felt obliged to admit
that among the indifferent matters some like health
were desirable, while others like disease were to be re-
jected. Chrysippus declared it to be madness not to
desire health, wealth, and absence of pain, and an incurable illness appeared sufficient reason for suicide.
Zeno hanged himself on account of a broken finger.[6]

It is obvious that the philosophers' high valuation
of health was shared by the physicians. The Hippocratic writer of the book *On Diet* stated: "Without
health nothing is of any use, not money nor anything

5. *Lyra Graeca*, III, 400–402.
6. The testimonies to these views in E. Zeller, *Die Philosophie
der Griechen in ihrer geschichtlichen Entwicklung* (4th ed. 1909),
Vol. III, Part I, 219.

else."[7] And the Alexandrian physician Herophilos expressed this view still more strongly in the sentence: "When health is absent, wisdom cannot reveal itself, art cannot become manifest, strength cannot fight, wealth becomes useless and intelligence cannot be applied."[8]

The physicians had an explanation for health. Health, they believed, was a condition of perfect equilibrium. When the forces (*dynameis*) or humors or whatever constituted the human body were perfectly balanced, man was healthy. Disturbed balance resulted in disease. This is still the best general explanation we have. Whether medicine thinks in terms of humors, vital forces, or physics and chemistry makes little difference. Health appears as a perfectly balanced condition.

The followers of Pythagoras, whose school had much more the character of a religious order than of a philosopher's school, endeavored to preserve the balance of health by leading a pure life and by subjecting themselves to a specific diet and practices. If illness occurred they sought medicine and music to restore the balance. Medicine and music were highly cultivated in their schools, whose influence upon further medical developments soon became apparent.

Attic education, the *Enkyklios Paideia*, including grammar, music, and gymnastics, tended to develop a harmonious, well-balanced individual, and palaestra

7. Peri diaites, Littré, VI, 604.
8. In Sextus Empiricus, *Adversus mathematicos,* II, 50; see Edelstein, *loc. cit.,* p. 268.

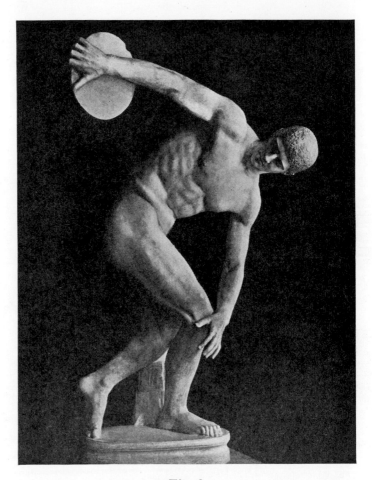

Fig. 9.

Discobolos.

Greek athletics.

and gymnasium became the experimental fields of physicians.

From the fifth century B.C. on, and throughout its course, Greek medicine was never exclusively curative medicine. The preservation of health seemed from the very beginning the more important task and in the fifth century physicians devoted a great deal of thought to problems of hygiene.

To the Hippocratic physician diet was the most important therapy, and dietetics therefore were highly developed. Drugs were given chiefly to intensify diets, and the knife was resorted to only when all other means failed. If appropriate diet was the chief method to cure disease, it seemed obvious that faulty diet was the principal cause of disease. The word diet, however, had a much broader meaning in antiquity than today. It implied a man's whole mode of living.

And so the Hippocratic physicians and their followers studied how a man should live in order to maintain his health. And they came to the conclusion that it was impossible for a man to remain in perfect health unless he organized his entire life for such a purpose. This attitude is illustrated by an extraordinarily interesting document, a fragment from a book on hygiene written by one of the most talented fourth-century physicians, Diocles of Karystos.[9] It describes a day spent in what the physicians considered a hygienic way. The text is too long and too detailed to be

9. Oribasius, ed. Bussemaker and Daremberg, III, 168 ff.

rendered literally and the following is a mere abstract and paraphrase:

The cultivation of health begins with the moment a man wakes up. This should as a rule be when the food he ate the previous day has already moved from the stomach to the bowels. A young or middle-aged individual should soon before sunrise take a walk of about 10 stadia, in the summer however of only 5, and older men will take a shorter walk in winter as well as in summer. After awakening one should not arise at once but should wait until the heaviness and torpor of sleep have gone. After arising one should rub neck and head thoroughly in order to overcome the stiffness caused by the pillow. Then the time has come to rub the whole body with some oil. Those who are not accustomed to empty their bowels immediately after arising should perform this rubbing before the evacuation, while others will do it after the evacuation but before undertaking anything else. . . . Thereafter one shall every day wash face and eyes with the hands using pure water. One shall rub the gums in order to strengthen the teeth or shall simply rub the teeth inside and outside with the fingers using some fine peppermint powder and cleaning the teeth of remnants of food. One shall anoint nose and ears inside, preferably with well-perfumed oil. . . . The head is a part that requires a great deal of care such as rubbing, unction, washing, combing, and close shaving. One shall rub and anoint the head every day but wash it and comb it only at intervals. . . . After such a morning toilet people who are obliged or choose to work will do so, but people of leisure will first take a walk. Long walks before meals evacuate the body, prepare it for receiving food, and give it more power for digesting it. Moderate and slow walks after meals mix foods, drinks and gases contained in the body. . . . After the walk it is good to sit down and to attend to private affairs until the time arrives when one has to think of caring for

the body. Young people and those who are accustomed to
exercise or who need it should go to the gymnasium. For
older and weaker people it is better to go to the bath or to
some other warm place to be anointed. For people of that
age if they have a gymnasium exclusively for their own use
a moderate rubbing and light exercise are sufficient. . . .
After such physical exercise it is time for breakfast which
in summer should consist of white barley groats with aro-
matic white wine well mixed with some honey and water—
or some other gruel that does not produce flatulence, is
nourishing and easy to digest. Those who do not care for
such foods shall take cold bread for breakfast. In addition
to that, one shall eat some boiled vegetable such as gourds
or cucumber, prepared simply. One shall drink white wine
and water until the thirst is quenched but before eating one
should drink water in large quantity if one is thirsty, otherwise less. Soon after breakfast one should go to sleep in a
shady or cool place well protected from wind. After the
siesta one can attend to private affairs, take another walk
and go to the gymnasium. After having exercised and being
covered with dust it is good for strong young people to have
a cold bath. Older and weaker people, on the other hand,
shall be anointed and rubbed gently and shall then have a
hot bath. A general rule is that one should never or only
rarely wash the head with hot water. . . . The chief meal
is to be taken when the body is empty and does not contain
any badly digested residue of food. Dinner should be taken
in summer soon before sunset and consist of bread, vegetables and barley cake. Dinner begins with raw vegetables,
with the exception of cucumber and horseradish, for these
are vegetables that should be eaten toward the end of the
meal. Boiled vegetables are eaten in the beginning of
the meal. Other dishes are cooked fish and meats, kid or lamb
meat shall be preferably from very young animals, pork
from middle-aged pig, and as far as birds are concerned one
shall eat chicken, partridge, or pigeon. All must be cooked

simply. . . . Before dinner one shall drink water and continue to drink it some time afterwards. Lean people shall drink dark and thick wine and after the meal white wine. Fat people shall drink white wine all the time, and they all shall drink their wine with water. Fruits from trees are of little use, but if one takes them in moderate quantities before the meals they do relatively little harm. . . . After dinner lean and flatulent people who do not digest well should go to sleep at once while others will take a short and slow walk before going to sleep. It is good for everybody to lie on the left side first as long as the food is still in the region of the stomach, but when the abdomen has become soft one should turn to the right. It is not good for anybody to sleep on the back.

This passage from Diocles' book gives a splendid picture of what the physicians of the period considered the ideal mode of living—one devoted to the preservation of health in which nutrition and evacuation, exercise and rest were perfectly balanced. It was an individual regimen taking sex, age, constitution, and the seasons, into careful consideration. A tremendous amount of research was done by Greek physicians on the influence of physical and nutritional factors on the human body, and their writings are full of splendid observations.

But it was perfectly obvious that very few people could afford to lead such a life. It was a regime for the wealthy few, for a small upper class leading a life of leisure, a class produced and supported by an economy in which all manual labor was performed by slaves. It was an aristocratic hygiene and one that was concerned with the body alone.

But what about those who had to work or chose to work, who were busy in politics, in science and learning, and in trade? The physicians had rules of conduct for them also. The Hippocratic writer of Book III, *On Diet*, mentioned above, devoted a long chapter to "the mass of people who drink and eat what they happen to get, who are obliged to work, and to travel by land and sea in order to make a living, who are exposed to unbecoming heat and unwholesome cold and who otherwise lead an irregular life."[10] All they can do is to remember the season in which they happen to be and try to adapt their meals, exercises, and sex life to the season as well as they can. It is little enough. They are people who "by necessity must lead a haphazard life and who, neglecting all, cannot take care of their health."

Nothing is said about the slaves, the farmers, and small artisans. There was no hygiene for them. They had no choice of food, no gymnastics. Regulation of work and rest was beyond their control. A really healthy life was accessible only to the rich and leisured class.

These views of the Hippocratic physicians and their followers did not remain unopposed and Plato was one of the first to attack them. The perpetual care for one's health appeared to him as just another disease. In a well-regulated state everyone has a function to fulfil. Nobody has time to be sick all his life under the pretence of attending to his health. This is

10. Littré, VI, 594–604.

perfectly obvious in the case of artisans but not so apparent in the case of the rich.[11]

The great social changes that occurred in the Hellenistic age reduced considerably the number of people who could lead a life of idleness. In principle the physicians still clung to their hygienic views, but they had to make concessions to the realities of life. And this was still more the case in the Roman period.

The Roman of wealth was a man of action, farmer, administrator, statesman, and soldier. Greek hygiene seemed useless and effeminate not only to men of Cato's type. The opposition to traditional hygiene became more and more articulate. Plutarch in the first century A.D. voiced it unmistakably in his *Advice About Keeping Well*, an essay which is full of common sense:

For health is not to be purchased by idleness and inactivity, which are the greatest evils attendant on sickness, and the man who thinks to conserve his health by uselessness and ease does not differ from him who guards his eyes by not seeing, and his voice by not speaking. For a man in good health could not devote himself to any better object than to numerous humane activities. Least of all is it to be assumed that laziness is healthful, if it destroys what health aims at; and it is not true either that inactive people are more healthy. For Xenocrates did not keep in better health than Phocion, nor Theophrastus than Demetrius, and the running away from every activity that smacked of ambition did not help Epicurus and his followers at all to attain their much-talked-of condition of perfect bodily health. But we ought, by attention to other details, to preserve the natural

11. *Republic* 3, 406c.

constitution of our bodies, recognizing that every life has room for both disease and health.[12]

The physicians began to express similar views. Celsus even went so far as to declare that a healthy man needed no special diet and no medical advice at all. Only weak individuals had to devote some attention to their bodies.

And gradually the concept of health broadened. While before it had been chiefly physical, it now was extended to include mental health. It was the Romans who expressed the wish *ut sit mens sana in corpore sano* and thus coined a slogan for centuries to come.

Oribasius in his great compilation has preserved a fragment on hygiene from the works of the philosopher Athenaeus which is a perfect gem. It is a document not only of physical but also of mental hygiene and I cannot resist the temptation to quote a few passages from it:

Little children who have been weaned must be permitted to live comfortably and playfully. They must be left in peace and when you exercise them do it with little jokes. They must be given very light food in moderate quantity, for people who stuff them with rich food after weaning pervert their nutrition and hinder their growth since their nature is weak still. . . . From the age of six or seven years boys and girls must be entrusted to gentle and humane teachers. Those who attract the children and in their teaching use persuasion and encouragement and praise them often, have better results and stimulate their zeal much more. The children love such teaching and feel at ease. Now relaxation

12. *De tuenda sanitate praecepta* 135, II, 280. Loeb Classical Series.

and a joyful mind contribute a great deal to good nutrition. Those masters, however, who nag and reprimand the children bitterly make their character servile and fearful, and make them loathe the subject of their teaching. They force them to learn by beating them and expect them to remember things while they are beaten when they have lost their presence of mind. It is not necessary either to bother the children the whole day long with instruction. On the contrary the greater part of the day should be devoted to play. Indeed we find even among robust mature people that the body weakens if they study without interruption. Children of twelve years already must follow courses in grammar and geometry and must exercise their bodies. But it is necessary that they have reasonable and experienced tutors so that they come to know the right measure and time for food, exercise, bath, sleep, and other details of the regimen. Most people pay a high price for their grooms and select careful and experienced people, while to teach their children they take individuals without experience who already have become useless . . .[13]

Mystics, such as the followers of the Neo-Platonic school, began to disregard care of the body and to concentrate their attention on the soul, but the physicians moved in another direction. Rome had conquered Greece materially but Greek culture had subjugated Rome. Gone were the old Roman virtues of republican days. Imperial Rome looked back to Greece. To the men living in the second century A.D. the fifth century B.C. appeared as the Golden Age. Romans endeavored to live like Greek gentlemen, watching their diet, exercising in the palaestra, spending their days

13. Oribasius, ed. Bussemaker and Daremberg, III, 161 ff.

in luxurious thermae. And the physicians encouraged
them. Galen, although an eclectic, considers himself a
disciple of the divine Hippocrates. In his voluminous
book *On Hygiene* old Hippocratic views are clearly
reflected:

Those who on account of ambition or other passions have
chosen a life of action that leaves them little time for the
care of the body, voluntarily serve evil lords. It is useless to
try to teach them what the best care of the body is. He,
however, who is totally free, by destiny and determination,
he alone can be shown how he may live in the best possible
health and be sick only rarely, and how he may get old most
gracefully.[14]

This sounds like a familiar tune. And in the same
chapter Galen distinguishes four types of men in re-
spect to health. By far the best is the one who has a
perfect constitution and leads a totally independent
life. Next follows one whose organism is defective but
whose life is free. The third type is represented by a
man who has a perfect constitution but lives in servi-
tude. Last, and worst of all, is a sickly body combined
with an unfree life. Freedom from passion, and economic independence were to Galen the chief prereq-
uisites of health, more important than good physical
constitution because it seemed impossible to lead a
life of health without complete independence.

The road was closed. Health and hygiene again
were a privilege of the leisure class. The working class
did not count. Labor was cheap as long as imperial

14. Ed. Kühn, VI, 82–83.

wars provided a constant supply of man power. And
when the empire was pacified, conditions had changed
and the institution of slavery was challenged.

The Greek concept of health was onesided, and
hygiene was limited in its application. It was the concept of a sensual people who had discovered the beauty
of the human body and worshiped it.

Christianity reacted against these views. The people to whom the new religion addressed itself had no
hygiene. They did not exercise or anoint themselves.
The thermae were not for them and they ate what
they could get. They were working people. Christianity did not recognize a leisure class that lived on
the labor of others. In the new religion work became
an ethical postulate. He who would not work, neither
should he eat. And the constant care of the body
seemed utterly ridiculous. What is a beautiful woman
if not a mere bag filled with excrements? Pagan hygiene cannot preserve health. It is the soul that
counts. Everybody is sick without Christ. Not diets
nor exercises are needed, but baptism is the bath that
gives health. The water of baptism is medicinal
water,[15] a healing remedy.[16] Therefore all heathen are
sick, whatever their hygiene may be, and the Church
is the hospital to treat them.[17]

This was a concept of health totally different from
Greek views. It was a purely spiritual concept, which
emphasized health of the soul, not of the body. A

15. *Aqua medicinalis,* Tertullian, de baptismo 1.
16. *Paionion pharmakon,* Clemens, Paedog. I, 6, 29.
17. See Adolf Harnack, *Medicinisches aus der ältesten Kirchengeschichte* (Leipzig, 1892).

beautiful soul could reside in a sick body, and a man could be a wreck physically and yet enjoy perfect health. Such health was not the privilege of a few. It was available to all, could be attained and preserved by whoever followed the precepts of Christ.

Ancient hygiene was violently opposed to this view, at least in its exaggerated form. One could not serve the body and God at the same time. But, just as the Church gradually reconciled itself to Hellenistic medicine, in the same way elements of ancient hygiene were admitted in the course of time. Was not the body the vessel of the soul created by God to serve him? Whoever wilfully destroyed it sinned. It became the Christian duty to consult the physician in case of need and to follow his prescriptions. Physician and medicine were considered secondary aids in the preservation of life. The primary cause was God. According to Gratian the Christian was not obliged to live *medicinaliter*, following the precepts of hygiene, *quia sanis omnia sana*, because to the healthy everything is wholesome, but he sins if knowingly and without sufficient reason he takes or does something which might make him sick or even destroy him.[18]

And since the body was to be preserved, as vessel of the soul, there was room for hygiene in the Middle Ages, too. It was derived from two main sources. Old pagan customs survived. Tacitus reports that the German people were fond of bathing and so we find

18. See Paul Diepgen, *Die Theologie und der ärztliche Stand* (Berlin-Grunewald, 1922), where the various passages are indicated.

that the bath played an important part throughout
the Middle Ages. In the spring, to celebrate the res-
urrection of nature, men and women bathed in wooden
tubs, sang, and drank wine. To those of us who live in
well-heated, evenly ventilated, and well-lighted houses
it is difficult to visualize the hardships that winter
brought upon our ancestors. Even the homes of the
rich were cold and dark, and to the poor winter meant
endless suffering. The advent of spring, therefore,
was a tremendous relief, to be celebrated in many
ways. The May bath was one of these old rituals that
had survived from pagan days. A new man came out
of the water—cleansed of the impurities of winter.

Another old custom: the guest in the manor was
welcomed with a hot bath to which sometimes rose
petals had been added. Fair maidens waited on him.
The monastery in the early Middle Ages already had
its bathroom for friars and pilgrims. Ekkehard IV,
the chronicler of Saint Gall, tells the whimsical story
of a lame Italian traveler who sought the hospitality
of the cloister. Following the custom, he was led to a
bathtub into which the friar poured hot water. This
was apparently too hot because soon the pilgrim began to yell in his mother tongue, "Cald, cald est!"
The Germanic friar understood that the water was
too cold and poured still hotter water until the half-
boiled guest forgot his lameness and jumped out of
the tub.[19]

The public bathhouse was a permanent institution

19. See Conrad Brunner, *Über Medizin und Krankenpflege im
Mittelalter in schweizerischen Landen* (Zürich, 1922), p. 49.

in the medieval city. It was licensed by the authorities
and provided both steam and water baths. On Satur-
days, or several times in the week, it was announced
all over town that the bath was hot. People from all
walks of life came, sweated, whipped themselves with
switches, made hot and cold ablutions, had their hair
cut and washed, had cupping glasses applied if some
old rheumatic pain bothered them. If a lady had a
pimple on her nose, the bathhouse was the place where

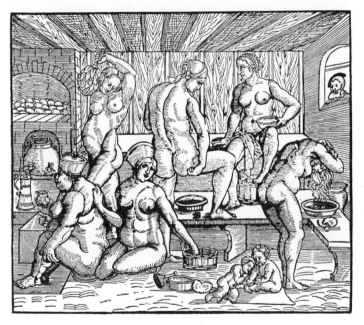

Fig. 10.

Medieval Bathhouse.

Woodcut by Hans Sebald Beham.

she could get advice. The owner of the house was a barber; he practiced minor surgery and was an expert in matters of cosmetics. He often had more experience in the treatment of skin diseases than the learned physician. He was the hygienic adviser of the people and the "beautician" of the medieval city. The bathhouse was the hygienic center of the town until syphilis began to plague Europe at the end of the fifteenth century, whereupon it became a center of infection and was gradually abolished.

The sweat and steam bath can be traced far back in history. It was known and was used for hygienic and curative purposes by primitive tribes all over the globe, particularly in the north. It was developed by the Romans, spread to the East, and came back to the West as the Turkish bath. It became an institution of the Russian village.

The medieval literature *de conservanda valetudine*, on the preservation of health, was derived from Greek and Roman sources. It consisted of reminiscences of the highly developed dietetics of classical days. The original works of the Hippocratic writers and of Galen were too long and too complicated for the period. Short treatises were needed setting forth brief hygienic rules that could be applied without undue trouble. In the fourth century A.D. such treatises were compiled in Greek and they were translated into Latin in the sixth century. They were anonymous or pseudonymous, carrying the name of some ancient sage or great physician. Two such short dietetic treatises were composed as epistles, and the fiction was that

they had been written by Hippocrates, one to Mae-
cenas and the other to a king Antiochus. Their great
popularity is evidenced by the large number of manuscripts preserved.[20] In a few pages they give advice
on how to live in the various seasons. Similar equally
brief texts provided short hygienic rules for the
months of the year. In the sixth century a physician
at the court of Theodoric, Anthimus, wrote a treatise
on the hygienic significance of various foodstuffs. It
was dedicated to a Frankish king, Theuderich. Ab-
stracts from various ancient writers were published
as separate treatises. All monastic rules had articles
regulating the periods of work and rest, prescribing
the number of meals and of dishes, frequently with
special regulations concerning friars of weak constitution.

Literature on hygiene was scanty in the early
Middle Ages but was common enough to preserve the
memory of ancient dietetics and to supply rules of
conduct to those who sought them.

Conditions changed in the twelfth century when
ancient literature became available through the me-
dium of translations from the Arabic. A Spanish Jew
converted to Christianity, John of Toledo, wrote in
Arabic a treatise on hygiene that was to become extremely popular. In order to make it more authorita-
tive he published it as a letter of Aristotle to Alexander the Great. The text was translated into Latin and

20. They were transmitted and are published with the book *De
Medicamentis* of Marcellus, *Corp. Med. Lat.* (Leipzig and Berlin,
1916), vol. V.

thence into the vernaculars. The Alexander letter
established a definite style. From then on the medieval
treatise on hygiene was as a rule a *regimen sanitatis,*
addressed to a person of high rank, advising him how
to live in order to preserve his health. It often pictured a day spent in the manner most becoming to
health, very much as Diocles had done. And what was
good for a king was good for a person of lower rank.

A large number of similar treatises were written
from the twelfth to the fifteenth centuries, in Latin
and vernacular languages. Whoever had a body-
physician urged him to write such a regimen, and
special treatises were composed, giving hygienic advice to people who had to travel over land or seas.

Undoubtedly the most popular book on hygiene
not only in the Middle Ages but of all times was the
Regimen Sanitatis Salernitanum. Few medical books
have had such wide distribution and have lived for
such a long time. Composed in the thirteenth century,
it gained its wide reputation because it was—rightly
or not—connected with the famous school of Salerno,
because it was written in verse so that it could be
memorized easily and, last but not least, because of
its sound common sense and keen sense of humor. The
introductory verses illustrate this:

> The Salerne Schoole doth by these lines impart
> All health to Englands King, and doth advise
> From care his head to keepe, from wrath his heart,
> Drinke not much wine, sup light, and soone arise,
> When meate is gone, long sitting breedeth smart:
> And after-noone still waking keepe your eyes.

When mov'd you find your selfe to Natures Needs,
Forbeare them not, for that much danger breeds,
Use three Physicions still; first Doctor Quiet,
Next Doctor Merry-man, and Doctor Dyet.[21]

It was an ideal manual for the people. There was hardly a situation that did not call for the quotation of some verses from this *Regimen*. How very much alive the text was is best illustrated by the fact that additions were constantly being made to it. Early manuscripts have a few hundred verses while some later editions number several thousand. The temptation to add to such a text was irresistible. Over one hundred manuscripts are preserved and there must be around five hundred printed editions.[22] The book was commented upon endless times, first in the thirteenth century by Arnald of Villanova, one of the leading physicians and medical writers of the period. In the following centuries whoever had a message to convey in matters of personal hygiene put it down in a commentary to the *Regimen Sanitatis Salernitanum*. As late as the nineteenth century, in 1880, a new edition was published in Paris, with a new commentary the purpose of which was not to explain the text historically but to add the experiences of modern medicine. The history of personal hygiene from the thirteenth to the nineteenth centuries could be writ-

21. *The School of Salernum, Regimen Sanitatis Salernitanum,* The English Version by Sir John Harington [1607] (New York, 1920), p. 75.
22. They are listed but by no means completely in L. Choulant, *Handbuch der Bücherkunde für die ältere Medicin* (Leipzig, 1841), p. 264 ff.

ten by merely discussing the various editions of this unusual text.

I have devoted so much space to medieval hygiene in order to show that in spite of the Christian emphasis on spiritual health, physical health was by no means neglected. It seemed desirable at all times. It is true that the health of the soul stood in the foreground and if it conflicted with physical health the body had to be sacrificed. Salvation was the purpose of life. But the realities of life were strong enough to force a compromise.

Looking back we can say that the Greek concept of health was primarily physical and that Greek hygiene was aristocratic. The Christian concept of health, on the other hand, was primarily spiritual and Christian hygiene was catholic, addressing itself to all. The synthesis of both, the development of a concept which would embrace physical and mental health without compromise, the revival, general adoption, and democratization of the *mens sana in corpore sano* of Juvenal—this ideal became the program of the ensuing centuries.

The process was slow, however, and the fulfilment of this program is far from accomplished. Little progress was achieved in the period of the Renaissance. Where the state power was strong, as in Elizabethan England, urban sanitation was improved following a trend that began in the fourteenth century after the ravages of the Black Death. The Reformation had a sobering influence upon the people. Luther had sound views about health and so, among the philosophers, had Montaigne.

Humanism, as a whole, was a spiritual and aristocratic movement. Its educational ideal was the *homo Ciceronianus* of Quintilian and centuries of monastic scholarship had also contributed to favor intellectual education at the expense of physical development.

Health conditions remained appallingly bad for a very long time. The brilliant court of Louis XIV was filthy and perfumes were needed to cover the stench emanating from unwashed bodies. Simple craftsmen of a medieval city had been far cleaner than were the noblemen in the seventeenth and even eighteenth centuries.

More than once conflicts occurred between the desire to keep the people in good health and fiscal needs. In the first half of the eighteenth century the consumption of gin increased tremendously in England.[23] It was encouraged by Parliament because it created a market for the farmers and brought revenues to the state. The result was that there was one tavern in London for every six houses and that alcoholism increased considerably. The same happened with tobacco. It was Richelieu's idea to make the use of tobacco a source of revenue for the state.[24] Other countries learned the lesson very quickly and today the tobacco industry has developed to such an extent that

23. Sir George Newman, *The Rise of Preventive Medicine* (London, 1932), p. 158.
24. Corti, *A History of Smoking* (London, 1931), p. 149 ff.

few countries could afford to suppress it in spite of
the obvious harm it does to the people's health.

The eighteenth century marks a turning point in
the history of public health. The importance of
health, both physical and mental, for the individual
and society was fully recognized and great efforts
were made to promote it by applying the scientific
and social means available at the time. The very
powerful health movement of the eighteenth century
shows two totally different trends, both determined
by definite political philosophies.

One of them took its origin in the philosophy of enlightened despotism. In the absolutist, autocratic
state the monarch was to the subjects what the father
was to his children. He was responsible for them and,
knowing what was good for them, ordered what they
should do so as to keep well. The absolutist state recognized the protection of the people's health as one
of its obligations, which was to be met by administrative measures. Laws and police regulations prescribed
what people should do and avoid to maintain or restore their health. The administration of public health
became a police function.

The internal security of the State is the aim of the general
science of police. A very important part thereof is the science that teaches us to handle methodically the health of
human beings living in society and of those animals they
need to assist them in their labors and for their sustenance.
Consequently we must promote the welfare of the population by means which will enable persons cheerfully and for
lengthy periods to enjoy the advantages which social life

can offer them. . . . Medical police, therefore, like the science of police in general, is a defensive art, is a doctrine whereby human beings and their animal assistants can be protected against the evil consequences of crowding too thickly upon the ground; and especially it is an art for the promotion of their bodily welfare in such a way that without suffering unduly from physical evils, they may defer to the latest possible term the fate to which, in the end, they must all succumb. How strange it is that this science, which day by day grows more essential to our race, should still be so little cultivated. . . . This may be due to the fact that only of late have people begun to realize the value of a human being, and to consider the advantage of the population.

The man who wrote these lines in 1779, Johann Peter Frank, was one of the chief exponents of this health movement. Born in the Palatinate, he grew up in that borderland between French and German civilization and spent all his life in the service of various rulers, in Germany, Austria, Italy, Poland, and Russia. Napoleon tried to lure him to Paris. He treated patients, reorganized hospitals, taught students, and instructed monarchs how to protect the health of their subjects. In Pavia he once gave a brilliant address in which he denounced poverty as the chief cause of disease. And throughout his life he worked on one great book that was published in six volumes from 1779 to 1817 under the title *System einer vollständigen medicinischen Polizey*. In this book Frank investigates and discusses the life of man from the moment of conception to the moment of death, as it evolves in its physical and social environment. He examines the factors that threaten health and recommends methods of counteracting them. His approach to public health is as broad as it can be. Man is a social being and in the causation of disease social factors are just as important as physical factors. He goes so far, for instance, as to examine the influence of the theater on the people's health.

Frank was a staunch supporter of the authoritarian state. His aim was to promote health through legislation and to enforce it through state organs. But he was well aware of limitations and in a significant passage he stated: "An intelligent police does not interfere with the privacy of the homes. If the police, this ruler of people, let itself be misused for spying, it degenerates and becomes the tyrant of human societies, and it disturbs the public order which it is called upon to protect."[25]

There was another totally different trend in the health movement of the eighteenth century. The philosophy of the Enlightenment was its background. It did not call upon the state for the protection of health but addressed itself to the individual. The state was corrupted, was an instrument of tyranny and oppression. Nothing good could be expected from it. Man, on the other hand, was good and reasonable by nature. He suffered from lack of knowledge, was unhappy because he was not enlightened, and sick because he was ignorant. Civilization had corrupted him and removed him from nature, from the natural condition of health and happiness. Education and en-

25. Frank, *System einer vollständigen medicinischen Polizey,* III, 957.

lightenment were needed in matters of health and hygiene.

Jean Jacques Rousseau was one of the exponents of this trend. But long before him John Locke in *Some Thoughts Concerning Education* [1693] had formulated a program of physical and mental health through education:

A Sound Mind in a sound Body, is a short, but full Description of a happy State in this World. He that has these two, has little more to wish for; and he that wants either of them, will be but little the better for anything else. Men's Happiness or Misery is most part of their own making. He, whose Mind directs not wisely, will never take the right Way; and he, whose Body is crazy and feeble, will never be able to advance in it. . . . And I think I may say, that of all the Men we meet with, nine Parts of ten are what they are, good or evil, useful or not, by their Education. 'Tis that which makes the great Difference in Mankind.

Since education seemed so all-important, great attention was given to the child, who was closer to nature, and still innocent. But, left to the care of nurses and tutors who had no understanding of its needs, the child soon lost its health and happiness. Emphasis was laid on the fact that the child is not a miniature adult, but a developing human being which has a physical and mental life of its own. Mothers were urged to nurse their children themselves. Century-old practices such as the tight swaddling of infants were denounced as injurious to health. In 1741 Nicolas Andry wrote *L'Orthopédie ou l'art de prévenir et de corriger dans les enfants les difformités du corps*, a

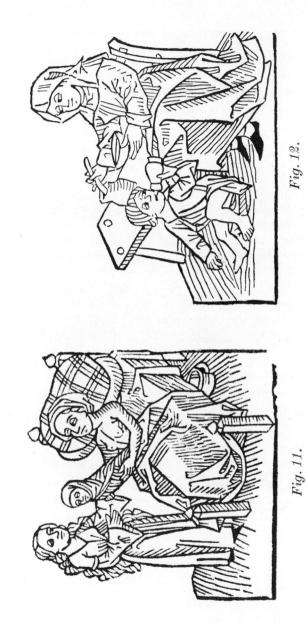

Fig. 11.

Swaddling the Infant.

Fig. 12.

Feeding the Infant.

Both from Heinrich Louffenberg's *Versehung des Leibs*, 1491.

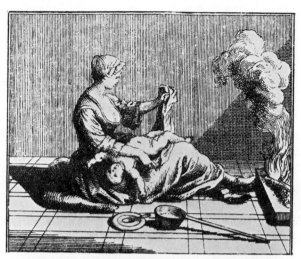

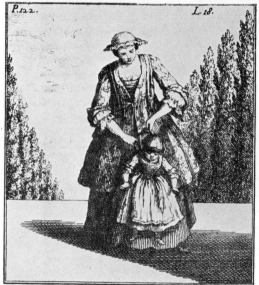

Fig. 13.

The Incorrect Handling of Children.

From Andry's *Orthopédie*, 1741.

book that coined the term orthopedics and in which
the author demonstrated that many deformities were
due to the wrong handling of children. In 1760 Jean
Charles des Essartz published a *Traité de l'éducation
corporelle des enfants en bas âge* which had the characteristic subtitle of *Réflexions pratiques pour pro-
curer une meilleure constitution aux citoyens,* a book
which Rousseau used extensively when he wrote his
novel *Émile* which was published in 1762.

In the following years a great many books and
pamphlets were written for the purpose of educating
the people in matters of health and one of the most
popular was the *Catechism of Health* of Bernhard
Christoph Faust, published in 1794.[26] It is a delight-
ful document, full of sound common sense, as true today in many respects as it was when it first came out.
Faust is a typical representative of the period, a German country doctor and small-town practitioner who
devoted his whole life to improving the people's health
and promoting general welfare. A dreamer, he advocated a league of nations, an ideal community em-
bracing all mankind, ruled by the same laws, enjoy-
ing the same liberties. He wrote a little book on mid-
wives and midwifery in rural districts and fought to
break some sexual taboos. The woman in labor should
bear her child in the sanctuary of the home, surrounded by the entire family. Then the children would
see what their origin is, accepting birth as a natural

26. H. E. Sigerist, "Faust in America," *Medical Life* (1934),
XLI, 192–207. On some further editions of Faust's "Catechism of
Health," *Bulletin of the Institute of the History of Medicine,* II
(1934), 392–401.

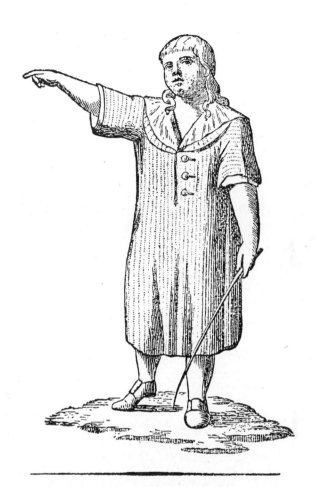

Wie vorſtehendes Kind gekleidet iſt, ſo ſollten
alle Kinder, ſowohl männlichen als weiblichen Ge-
ſchlechts, vom Anfange des dritten, bis zum Ende
des ſiebenten oder achten Jahrs gekleidet werden.

Fig. 14.

Bernhard Christoph Faust's Hygienic Dress for Children.

From *Gesundheits-Katechismus*, 1794.

process and not a mysterious operation. It would extinguish morbid curiosity and, as a result, innocence and peace would return among men.

In another study published in 1791, *How To Regulate the Sexual Instinct of Men and How To Render Men Better and Happier*, Faust came to the conclusion that wrong clothing of children was frequently responsible for sexual precocity, and he advocated a loose dress for children of both sexes. He was anxious to have it adopted officially and since the German governments were not responsive he had the book translated into French and presented it to the National Assembly in Paris. The revolutionary government of France, however, was busy with other problems.

Faust's most important contribution undoubtedly was his *Catechism of Health*. It was written for teachers, parents, and children as a manual of health education. It was translated into several languages, reprinted frequently, and it has been estimated that over 150,000 copies must have been sold within a few years. It was translated into English the year it came out and two American editions were printed, warmly recommended by Dr. Benjamin Rush and Dr. Hugh Williamson. The book was written as a catechism, in questions and answers. Its character and the underlying concept of health are best illustrated by quoting the first paragraphs:

Q. 1. Dear Children, to breathe, to live in this world, created by God, is it an advantage? Is it to enjoy happiness and pleasure?

A. Yes. To live is to enjoy happiness and pleasure; for life is a precious gift of the Almighty.

Q. 6. What is understood by a state of good health?

A. That the body is free from pains and infirmities, fulfills its duties cheerfully and with ease, and is always obedient to the soul.

Q. 7. How does he feel who enjoys health?

A. Strong; full of vigour and spirits; he relishes his meals; is not affected by wind and weather; goes through exercise and labour with ease, and feels himself always happy.

Q. 9. Can you children be merry and laugh, joke, and jump about, eat, drink, and sleep, when you are ill?

A. No. We can only do so when we are in good health.

OBSERVATION

If a child be present who was ill not long ago, the Master will take the opportunity of asking him the following question:—"You was ill; tell me did you feel yourself so happy, so easy as you do now?" To this a sensible child will answer, or will be taught to answer—"I found myself exceedingly ill, I could neither eat, drink, nor sleep; nothing afforded me pleasure or joy; I was full of anxiety and pains; but now restored to health; thanks be to God, I know it is the greatest good."

Q. 15. Is it sufficient if he take care of his own health?

A. No. It is also his duty to take care of the life and health of his fellow-creatures.

Q. 16. And what is the duty of parents towards their children?

A. They are bound to take the tenderest care of their health and life.

Faust was by no means alone. Wherever the spirit of the Encyclopedists had penetrated, doctors arose spreading the gospel of health enthusiastically. Numerous popular magazines were founded for the purpose.[27] All of them were short lived because the great health movement broke down. It did so for various reasons. The apostles of health of the type of Faust were humanitarians and idealists, who assumed that education was all-powerful and thus neglected economic factors. They told the people what they should eat in order to keep well and overlooked the fact that most people could not afford the recommended food. They addressed themselves primarily to the middle class, not to the peasants and city workers, most of whom could not read anyway.

Another factor which retarded developments was the dark political reaction that set in after the Napoleonic wars. Frank's last volume was published in 1817. It came too late. Most of his recommendations were never carried out. The bourgeoisie was growing rich and had no overwhelming interest in the public welfare. There was no break in continuity, to be sure. Books appeared like Christoph W. Hufeland's *Art of Prolonging Life*, first published in German in 1797, translated into eight languages, and reprinted constantly almost throughout the nineteenth century. Nevertheless, the health movement had lost its momentum and was not to recover until the emergency created by the Industrial Revolution.

The introduction of the steam engine into industry

27. See, for instance, Fridolin Lustenberger, *Schweizerische medizinisch-naturwissenschaftliche Zeitschriften von 1751–1871. Ihre Bedeutung und ihre Ziele* (Inaugural Dissertation, Zürich, 1927).

and the resulting industrialization of the Western World created a totally new situation. Factories provided employment for unskilled men, women, and children whose only property was their labor power. The new means of transportation made it possible to import food so that the population could increase beyond the capacity of the soil. Large masses of people were crowded in suburbs of cities, where they lived on starvation wages under appalling conditions, working endless hours unprotected against the new hazards of industry. In the working-class parishes of Saint John and Saint Margaret in London 5,366 families, or 26,830 individuals, lived in 5,294 rooms, and in Little Ireland, a district of Manchester, there was one toilet for every 120 inhabitants.[28]

When a worker was disabled or became unemployed in the course of one of the many crises, there was no other way open to him than to seek help under the Poor Laws, which meant virtual slavery.

Health conditions of the working population of England were atrocious. Hundreds of thousands died prematurely "from the effects of manufactures, civic states, and the intemperance connected with these states and occupations,"[29] and hundreds of thousands dragged on a miserable life crippled by disease.

This was a new situation, which could not be remedied through education, with health catechisms,

28. Friedrich Engels, *Die Lage der arbeitenden Klasse in England* (2d ed. 1848), p. 44 ff.
29. C. Turner Thackrah, *On the Effects of Arts, Trades, and Professions, and of Civic States and Habits of Living, on Health and Longevity* (1832), p. 5.

but required drastic measures. The seriousness of the problem was dramatically revealed when an epidemic of cholera invaded the country. People became aware that a sick working class is not only wasteful but also a menace to the rich. Therefore action was taken, coming from many sides and with different motivations. Humanitarianism characterized the efforts of social reformers and Utopian socialists of the type of Robert Owen. They felt indignant at the injustice of the existing order and strongly felt the disgrace of having such conditions in a country that claimed to be civilized. But, as Utopians, they believed that simply to demonstrate how much better conditions could be would suffice to improve matters, even in the teeth of a system of ruthless exploitation.

There was sound utilitarianism in the efforts of the government to revise the Poor Laws, a movement in which Edwin Chadwick played an important part. Chadwick, who became the pioneer of the English public health movement, was close to Jeremy Bentham. It was not a matter of philanthropy but in the interest of all to have a healthy working class. Chadwick seized the bull by the horns and endeavored not to relieve the effects of evil conditions but to remove their causes, economic, social, and physical. It was primarily due to him that the early English public health movement was so broad in its approach. His major crime in English eyes was that he believed in the greater efficiency of centralized administration.[30]

30. See Sir Arthur Newsholme, *Fifty Years in Public Health* (London, 1935). Iago Galdston, "Humanism and Public Health," *Bulletin of the History of Medicine,* VIII (July, 1940), 1032–1039.

And then—and this is probably one of the most important factors—there were the efforts of the working class itself. Health cannot simply be dispensed to the people. They must themselves want it and must fight for it. Militant unions were organized for the purpose of improving working and living conditions. Benefit societies were founded. The industrial workers lost their slave attitude, refused to accept conditions with fatalism, and struggled to improve them.

The nineteenth-century public health movement began in England because both the Industrial Revolution and its evil effects on health were felt there first. But wherever industries were developed similar effects resulted and called for similar remedies. Chadwick published his *Report on the Sanitary Condition of the Labouring Class* in 1842. In 1840 a French physician, Louis-René Villermé, published a report in two volumes on conditions among French textile workers.[31] But in 1807 the French prefect of police Dubois had already presented a report that exposed the appalling health conditions of the industrial population.[32] It was in France that Patissier in 1822 drew up a sound program for the improvement of conditions. Dangerous trades should be forbidden entirely or, if this proved to be impossible, only criminals sentenced to death and pardoned to hard labor should be allowed to work in them. Research should

31. *Tableau de l'état physique et moral des ouvriers employés dans les manufactures de coton, de laine et de soie* (Paris, 1840).

32. International Labour Office, *Occupation and Health: Encyclopaedia of Hygiene, Pathology and Social Welfare* (Geneva, 1934), II, 379.

be undertaken in order to improve working conditions and reduce health hazards of industry. Public baths should be made easily available to workers and, finally, workers disabled through their labor should be compensated and should have old-age insurance. It took a long time before these principles were generally accepted, but in 1822 France already had one hundred and twenty mutual benefit societies.

Germany in the first half of the century consisted of over thirty small and semifeudal states. Industry developed late and slowly. In 1837 there were only 419 stationary steam engines in Prussia, but then their number increased in the following 12 years to 1,444 and by 1849 Prussia had in addition 429 locomotives and 90 steamships. Health conditions were even worse than in England.

Health problems became so acute that in Germany, just as in England and France, action had to be taken. A powerful reform movement developed in the years preceding the Revolution of 1848.[33] Directed against bureaucracy, special privilege, and clerical obscurantism, it fought for a complete reorganization of health services. It was led by liberal physicians, and since the battle had to be fought in the political arena, doctors did not hesitate to enter the field of politics.

The head of the movement was Rudolf Virchow who later was to become Germany's outstanding pa-

33. See the excellent study of E. Ackerknecht, "Beiträge zur Geschichte der Medizinalreform von 1848," *Sudhoffs Archiv für Geschichte der Medizin,* XXV (1932), 61–109, 113–183.

thologist. He was born in 1821 and was young and
fiery in the revolutionary years. In 1847 an epidemic
of relapsing fever was devastating the industrial districts of Silesia. The government, under pressure of
public opinion, appointed a committee of investigation of which Virchow was a member. He soon came to
the conclusion that the causes of the epidemic were as
much social and economic as they were physical. His
report was a passionate indictment of the regime. The
remedy he recommended was prosperity, education,
and liberty, which can develop only on the basis of
"complete and unrestricted democracy." These were
unusual words in an epidemiological report, but they
are characteristic of the whole trend. Back in Berlin
Virchow founded in 1848 a new journal, *Die medizinische Reform*, which became the organ of the
movement. "The physicians," he wrote in the introductory article, "are the natural attorneys of the
poor, and social problems fall to a large extent within
their jurisdiction."

This great health movement is little known outside
of Germany. And yet when today, after almost one
hundred years, we read the numerous books and pamphlets written at the time, we find them incredibly
modern. They still have a message to carry. What
were the leading ideas and postulates?

"Medicine is a social science," wrote Virchow, the
pathologist, "and politics is nothing else but medicine
on a large scale."[34] The physician who lives in such
close touch with the people knows social conditions

34. *Die medizinische Reform*, p. 2.

better than anybody else and, being an expert in these matters, he must have a voice in government, if conditions are to be improved.

The goal is health for the people, for all the people, whether rich or poor. What are the means? Capital and labor must have equal rights; the living force of labor must no longer be subjected to dead capital. Only a free association of labor and capital can improve social conditions. This requires full-fledged democracy, equal rights for all. Education is needed and it must be free and available to all, even including free university education.

The people's health is a direct concern of government. This had been repeated in Germany since 1820, when L. Mende had written, "The State must protect health as its most precious property,"[35] and in 1848 it was formulated in the sentence, "The State representing the totality of all its members has the duty to care for their physical welfare and, therefore, has the duty to make provisions for the cultivation and maintenance of health and for the restoration of disturbed health conditions." Demands were made for public medical services for the indigents, for an increase in hospital facilities which would not only serve the people better but also raise the standard of medical care. The hospital was to be the center of medical practice. Voices were raised asking compensation for the loss of wages due to illness, and demanding sickness insurance financed by contributions from the workers

35. *Die Medizin in ihrem Verhältnis zur Schule, zu den Kranken und zum Staat* (Greifswald, 1820).

and from the propertied classes with municipal and state subsidies. Further postulates included the erection of a central Ministry of Health advised by a Physician's Parliament; the foundation of an Academy of Medicine to serve as a clearinghouse for medical research; uniform license, entitling physicians to practice in every German state; appointment of physicians to public offices on the basis of contests.

This was the Germans' National Health Program one hundred years ago.

In all these discussions the citizens' *right to health* was postulated more and more loudly. It was justified in a way which proves that the whole movement was by no means socialistic but a true middle-class liberal movement. The right to own property, even the means of production was not contested. S. Neumann, one of the most brilliant minds of the period, in his book *Public Health and Property*,[36] justifies the right to health in the following way. The state claims to be a state of property rights. Its purpose is to protect the people's property. Most people, however, possess nothing but their labor power, which depends entirely on their health. This is their only property and the state, therefore, has the duty to protect it and the people have the right to insist that their health, their only possession, be protected by the state.

The German Revolution of 1848 collapsed and with it the health movement declined. After having published ten numbers, Virchow had to discontinue his journal. In his last editorial he wrote:

36. *Die öffentliche Gesundheitspflege und das Eigentum* (Berlin, 1847).

We must wander through the desert and struggle. Our task
is an educational one. We must raise men able to fight the
battle of humanism. Further publication of our journal will
be useless because we have nothing more to expect from the
government. It is only left for us to accept the task: to edu-
cate the people concerning the problems of health, and to
assist them toward winning the final victory by continuously
providing for them new teachers. The medical reform which
we intended to bring about was a reform of science and society. We discussed its principles; even without the continua-
tion of our organ will they eventually be acknowledged.[37]

The great, forceful, and promising German health
movement with its far-reaching program had broken
down. Why? Chiefly because it was a movement of
liberal middle-class physicians *for* the people but
without the people. The people were never consulted.
They had no voice in all these deliberations. The people's health, however, is the concern of the people
themselves. They must want health. They must
struggle for it and plan for it. Physicians are merely
experts whose advice is sought in drawing up plans
and whose coöperation is needed in carrying them
out. No plan, however well devised and well inten-
tioned, will succeed if it is imposed on the people. The
war against disease and for health cannot be fought
by physicians alone. It is a people's war in which the
entire population must be mobilized permanently.

One of the tragedies of mankind is that most people
refuse to learn from the teachings of history, and that
mistakes are repeated over and over again.

37. *Die medizinische Reform,* p. 273 ff. Translation by Gertrude
Kroeger, *The Concept of Social Medicine* (Chicago, 1937), p. 12.

The German health movement did not mature, but the seed was sown—and some of the principles of 1848 were fulfilled after the unification of the German empire. Sickness insurance was introduced in 1883.

Wherever industries began to develop the same problems became acute, even in Tsarist Russia. An industrial development is impossible where the peasants are tied to the soil and have not the freedom to leave the land and join the factory. And so serfs were liberated in Russia in 1861. Factories cannot work if laborers are in ill health. And so Russia established a system of state medical services for the rural districts in 1864, and in 1866 a law was issued requiring factory owners to have one hospital bed available for every one hundred workers.

The establishment of conscript armies in most European countries during the nineteenth century brought a new factor into the attitude toward health. Nations now urgently needed a healthy and fit young generation to defend the country or to carry out imperialistic aims. And since the training of armies was in the hands of the government, the promotion of health automatically became a concern of the state. Athletics were a privilege of a small upper class in ancient Greece, a privilege of the nobility in the Middle Ages. In the eighteenth century philosophers recommended physical exercise as a method of education. In the nineteenth century governments and national interests encouraged athletics for military and disciplinary reasons. After the Napoleonic wars *Turnvereine*, or athletic clubs, were organized in Germany to prepare a healthy well-disciplined generation. They were highly political bodies, torchbearers of the country's national aspirations. The same was true of the *Sokol* movement founded in the 1860's in Slavic countries of central Europe and the Balkans, athletic organizations which became most active centers of pan-Slavism. When it became evident after the Treaty of Versailles that the world was marching toward still greater catastrophes than the World War, and new imperialisms became manifest, a race set in, not only in armaments but also in developing youth organizations whose purpose it was to prepare the new generation for the slaughter.

The great progress of medical science in the second half of the nineteenth and in the twentieth centuries forged new weapons for warding off disease and particularly for the control of communicable diseases. Bacteriology confirmed the hazy guesses of previous generations that infectious diseases were caused by living agents and revealed that certain diseases were due to the action of definite bacteria or other microorganisms. Accordingly, the protection of man against germs became one of the chief tasks of public health. It had always been assumed that drinking water should be pure, but bacteriology enabled us to control and measure the purity of water. Immunology indicated methods of building up resistance against definite diseases. Inoculation of smallpox was practiced successfully throughout the eighteenth century and vaccination was a great improvement in that it reduced the hazards considerably. The work of Pas-

teur, Koch, Behring, and others opened up new horizons, and diseases such as diphtheria, typhoid, cholera,
and lockjaw became preventable.

Bacteriology revealed external, biological causes
of diseases and, blinded by the great success of the
new science, physicians were often inclined to over-
look the social, economic, and individual factors that
are just as decisive in the genesis of disease. There is
no tuberculosis without tubercle-bacilli, but while
most people are exposed to infection, very few actually develop the disease. A low standard of living can
be as much responsible for the disease as the bacilli.

Even at the height of the bacteriological era, however, there were men who, like Pettenkofer in Munich,
were fully aware of the significance of the social environment, and others, like Rosenbach, Hueppe, and
Martius, who pointed out the importance of the con-
stitutional factor in the causation of disease. Pettenkofer, in his classical lectures on health conditions in
Munich,[38] successfully inaugurated the field of medical economics.

Sanitation and the protection of society against
communicable diseases are still a major function of
public health, but the field has broadened considerably in the last few decades. In the United States today only one tenth of the work carried out by public
health services is devoted to the traditional tasks and
nine tenths are devoted to new tasks, such as prenatal
and maternity care, infant welfare, school hygiene,

38. *Über den Wert der Gesundheit für eine Stadt* (Braun-
schweig, 1873).

treatment of venereal diseases, etc. Wherever private medicine proved unable to solve a problem, public services had to step in, in order to protect the people's health.

This long historical analysis has given us a clearer view of health and its significance for human welfare. Like the Romans and like John Locke, we think of health as a physical and mental condition. *Mens sana in corpore sano* remains our slogan. But we may go one step further and consider health in a social sense also. A healthy individual is a man who is well balanced bodily and mentally, and well adjusted to his physical and social environment. He is in full control of his physical and mental faculties, can adapt to environmental changes, so long as they do not exceed normal limits; and contributes to the welfare of society according to his ability. Health is, therefore, not simply the absence of disease: it is something positive, a joyful attitude toward life, and a cheerful acceptance of the responsibilities that life puts upon the individual.

It may seem farfetched to extend the concept of health into the social field. And yet there can be no doubt that an individual who is maladjusted socially does not possess the balance that constitutes health. A criminal who lives outside of society following rules of his own is like a malignant tumor governed only by its own metabolism. Both may seem healthy for a while, but ultimately the tumor destroys itself, and so with the criminal. He is sick and in need of a physician. Physical restoration is not the end of a medical

treatment. Since illness gives the patient a special position in society the cure is not complete before the
patient has been readjusted socially and enabled
either to resume his old position or adjust himself to
a new one. The goal of medicine is social and medicine
actually is a social science. The German physicians of
1848 were right.

Health, of course, is desirable today as it was in
former periods. It is one of our most precious posses-
sions and is a prerequisite for human welfare and
happiness. But it is more than desirable, it is necessary. A highly differentiated, highly specialized industrial society in which every member depends for
his welfare on the coördinated efforts of his fellowmen, has no room for unnecessary sickness but requires healthy members in order to function nor-
mally. A democracy in which the destiny of the
nation is the personal responsibility of every citizen
requires health.

We do not hesitate to accept the concept of man's
right to health or, more correctly, of man's right
fully to benefit from all known means for the protection and cultivation of health. We need no longer
justify health, as Neumann did, by declaring it to be
a form of property which the state is pledged to protect. If we believe that life, liberty, and the pursuit of
happiness are inalienable rights of man and that government is instituted to secure these rights, then we
must conclude that man has a right to health and is
entitled to having this right secured. Disease is a
threat to life, holding man in bondage and obstruct-

ing him in the pursuit of happiness. And when a
country establishes a constitution with the purpose of
promoting the general welfare, it thereby admits that
the health of the people is a direct concern of government.

If we recognize the right to health we are justified
in postulating a duty to health. This is a new attitude which has developed only recently, as a result of
a sharpening social consciousness. We mentioned ear-
lier that in several countries the venereal patient who
evades treatment is punishable and so is the soldier
who evades his duty by wilfully letting himself become sick. More and more we accept the view that
man has a civic duty to fulfil which requires health.

Health is not inevitable or obvious: it must be protected and cultivated, and this requires, first of all,
knowledge. The more we know about health and disease, the more effectively we can act. Scientific and
sociological research is, therefore, the source that
feeds all our actions. But knowledge alone is not
enough. In order to become effective it must be applied and this is only possible if it is shared by all the
people. Education, therefore, is all important. I must
repeat that the people's health is the concern of the
people themselves. They must be enlightened in matters of health. They must want it and take an active
part in its administration. And since the protection
of health is a task of great magnitude the people will
endeavor to fulfil it collectively through the state and
its organs. This is why health is a primary concern of
the people *and* of government. The physicians and

medical officers, those who have both general and expert knowledge in matters of health, are, therefore, best able to advise and guide the people of whom they are a part.

The state can protect society very effectively against a great many dangers, but the cultivation of health, which requires a definite mode of living, remains to a large extent an individual matter and is the result of education. It is no exaggeration to say that the school is one of the most important public health institutions. It must help the child to develop all his physical and mental faculties, to acquire health habits, and to build up that attitude toward life which is part of health. The school provides the ideal opportunity to have children under permanent medical control and to remedy in time defects due to heredity or environment. Health should be a subject of instruction in every grade from elementary school to university, and particular attention must be given to adolescent children in secondary schools at a period when asocial drives begin to manifest themselves. This is the moment when mental hygiene becomes particularly significant. Teachers must be thoroughly trained in health matters. The school medical officer does not know the individual children and sees them only at long intervals, while the teacher has the opportunity of watching them daily. He is the first to notice that something is wrong with a child, and he must bring him to the attention of the medical officer. If the school succeeded in nothing else but in developing healthy young people, it would have achieved a great

deal, and while many of them may later not be able to
lead a healthy life under the pressure of social and
economic conditions, still if they once have acquired
sound health habits they will at least live as well as
conditions permit.

The health program of every country can be sum-
marized in a few points. Such a program must provide:

1. Free education to all the people, including
   health education.
2. The best possible working and living conditions.
3. The best possible means of rest and recreation.
4. A system of health institutions and medical personnel, available to all, responsible for the people's health, ready and able to advise and help
   them in the maintenance of health and in its
   restoration when prevention has broken down.
5. Centers of medical research and training.

It is an ambitious program which has not yet been
fulfilled anywhere, but every civilized country is moving in that direction, some more rapidly, others more
slowly, and they all agree that health is one of the
most important factors in human welfare.

III. THE PHYSICIAN

THE study of history is not a luxury. History is one of the most powerful driving forces in our life. Unlike animals, we are conscious of the past, and the picture we carry in us of our history determines our actions to a very large extent, whether we are aware of it or not.

All professions have the tendency to glorify their own past. In antiquity medicine was believed to be of divine origin. It was Thoth who revealed the healing art to the Egyptians, Apollo to the Greeks, and the first physicians, Imhotep and Asklepios, were deified. Greek physicians traced their ancestry back to Asklepios, calling themselves Asklepiads, thus exalting their past.

We do exactly the same. We have in the course of time built a legendary, sentimental, and romantic history of our profession in which most physicians blindly believe. We assume that the physician was at all times a wise and worthy gentleman, highly respected in his community, sacrificing himself disinterestedly for the benefit of his patients. We have almost deified Hippocrates, of whom we know very little, or rather we have created a mythical Hippocrates who has nothing to do with the historical figure, in order to satisfy our romantic desire for an ancestor and a symbol.

We still require our young physicians to swear the Hippocratic Oath, and they do it in some awe. In so doing, they swear by pagan gods, in whom they do not believe, that they will not practice surgery, that they will share their livelihood with their teachers and adopt their sons. And yet the young doctors do not hesitate to practice surgery, even on patients suffering from the stone. And very few physicians have ever shared their income with their professors or adopted their sons. We reveal professional secrets when interests of society are involved. Our attitude toward abortion is determined by law, and we perform it whenever it is justified medically. That the physician should not injure his patients deliberately or have sexual intercourse with them should be pretty obvious. In the whole oath there is only one positive pledge: "In purity and in holiness I will guard my life and my art," and the purpose of the oath is to gain for the physician "reputation" (doxa). In a society which did not license its physicians a doctor was legitimized by his reputation.

Whoever swears the Hippocratic Oath is sure to commit perjury. Why then do we still swear it? Because it is old; because the name of Hippocrates is attached to it, and because generations of physicians have sworn it before us. In short, we do it because it fits into the sentimental picture we have made of our past.

I do not underestimate the great value of flags and symbols. We need them, but in order to be inspiring they must be true. It is not harmless to begin a career with an oath that we are sure to break. Since history molds the future and since the views we have of our past are so influential in determining our actions, it is perfectly obvious that untrue history must cause a great deal of harm. That there are so many misunderstandings among physicians today is, in my opinion, to a large extent due to the fact that many doctors have wrong views of history. They may be great and honest scientists, highly critical in their own field, but when it comes to history they seem to lose all critical faculty, to accept the most absurd statements and use them as arguments without even testing them. There is, of course, a personal element in the interpretation of historical data, just as there is in science, but historical research also has its rules which impose an iron discipline upon the historian.

Let us try in a realistic way to trace briefly the history of the physician's profession.[1]

The task has always been the same: to promote health by preventing illness and curing it. Every society required of its physician that he have knowledge, skill, devotion to his patients, and similar qualities. But his position in society, the tasks assigned to him, and the rules of conduct imposed upon him changed in every period. They were determined primarily by the social and economic structure of society and by the technical and scientific means available to medicine at the time.

The physician is by no means the only medical worker. Even in remote times he had assistants to

1. See H. E. Sigerist, "The Physician's Profession through the Ages," *Bulletin of the New York Academy of Medicine,* IX (1933), 2d ser., 661–676.

help him in his task, and this very important auxil-
iary medical personnel increased with every century
as medical knowledge became more diversified. In a
country like the United States more than a million
people are actively engaged in health work.

And then there is, and always has been, a great
deal of self-treatment. The overwhelming majority
of all cases of illness are never seen by the physician.
A great number of minor ailments—colds, coughs,
headaches, and stomach-aches—are treated by the
patient himself or by his relatives. This self-medica-
tion may follow principles of scientific medicine or
may be dictated by popular beliefs, superstitions, or
views forced upon the people by commercial interests.
This is the field where the patent medicine industry
finds such a flourishing market.

The physician, however, is the medical expert of
society. He knows more about health and disease than
other people. He has acquired his initial knowledge
by studying with masters who have passed on to him
the accumulated experience of centuries and the results of their own researches. He continues to learn
while practicing medicine. Observation, experience,
experimentation, and reasoning are the sources of his
knowledge. He satisfies his need for causality by de-
vising theories that explain the phenomena observed
and the results of his actions. Theories guide him in
his thinking and acting and are modified whenever
new observations call for it. A doctor thinks in the
concepts available in his time and this is why medical
theories have been magical or religious, philosophical

or scientific. The theory of the four humors was just
as true in antiquity as physico-chemical theories are
today. The physician of genius, the medical leader, is
not the man who thinks in terms totally different from
those of his contemporaries. If he did he would not be
understood, would have no influence and would possibly land in a lunatic asylum. The leader is the man
who, using the concepts of the day, moving with the
trends, is yet ahead of his time, anticipating the future, and thus drawing his contemporaries after him.
Medical theories are deeply rooted in the general civilization of a period and like general culture are the
result of material conditions.

The physician's success or failure, however, depends not only on his knowledge and skill. If society
is not willing or able to accept them, all his efforts are
in vain. The responsiveness of society is determined
by endless social, economic, religious, philosophic,
and political factors.

In primitive society the medicine man was and still
is sorcerer, priest, and physician in one. He acts as a
sorcerer when he fights witchcraft with magical
means, as a priest when he placates the gods or the
spirits of the deceased, and his function is that of a
physician in that he endeavors to cure sick people.
He is skilled in the interpretation of *omina*, knows
how to discover and punish a culprit, is familiar with
charms, and versed in the uses of herbs and physical
treatments. He can cure ailments and can make rain.
In some tribes shamanism is hereditary and son is initiated by father, or daughter by mother. In other

tribes children are marked for their future career by
the spirits at birth. A child born with a tooth or with
a caul or in an abnormal position must be a child of a
special kind. Or unusual happenings may indicate
the spirits' intentions. A child falls from a tree without being hurt: how could this be unless the child had
special protection? As apprentice to a shaman the
young man or woman learns the difficult craft. Each
is taught about the ways of the spirits, learns how to
communicate with them through prayers, rites, and
in ceremonial procedures. While in training the apprentice must, in many tribes, abstain from definite
foods, bring sacrifices, and sometimes even undergo
mutilations. Initiated at last, he becomes a shaman
himself and is invested with drum, amulets, and all
the insignia and tools of his craft.

In some agricultural tribes the medicine man is a
farmer like the other tribesmen and practices his art
only on special occasions. His remuneration is modest
and he remains poor like his fellows. In many other
tribes, however, he leads a life of his own, a lonely
life. His hut is outside the village. He is often rich,
because people pay him willingly, sometimes in advance, sometimes according to the gravity of the case,
success of the cure, or rank of the patient. He is regarded with awe, is respected and feared. Since he
knows how to counteract witchcraft, he obviously
knows also how to bewitch people, and he is frequently suspected.

He is often the bard of the tribe. Music and dances
are part of his ritual. He can tell many legends and

stories about the origin of the world. He is familiar
with the traditions of the tribe and passes them on to
his pupils. Also many shamans are psychopathic per-
sonalities.

We mentioned in a previous chapter that the basic
views of primitive medicine never died. They are still
alive and can be found as superstitions in our modern
society. In the same way the physician has never quite
freed himself of certain traits of the medicine man.

The structure of Babylonian society and the character of its science determined the physician's position. In a world in which all science was subordinate
to theology he was diviner and priest. We have already seen him, conjuring and exorcising evil spirits.
There is some evidence that surgeons were laymen,
possibly slaves of the priest-physician, but the sources
are scanty and do not allow definite conclusions.

Sources are plentiful when we come to ancient
Greece. The Hippocratic physician was a craftsman
like the shoemaker, the blacksmith, or the painter.
Like other craftsmen, he was trained through ap-
prenticeship. He selected a master, paid him a fee,
and spent a number of years with him in his work-
shop, the *iatreion*, or on tours. He assisted him in
mixing drugs or holding the patient who was operated on, and from him he learned to observe symptoms of disease and to evaluate them critically in
making a prognosis. He also learned how to prescribe
diets and drugs and how to perform operations, until
the day came when he was a master himself.

The number of physicians was small and only the

larger cities had doctors permanently in residence. When a city was anxious to have a physician settle down, it offered him an annual salary which was raised

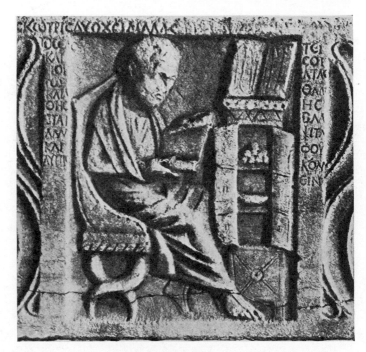

Fig. 15.

The Greek Physician.

Relief from a Roman sarcophagus.

through a special tax. This did not prevent him from accepting fees but it did guarantee him an income even in times when there was not much work.

Most places, however, were served by wandering physicians, for in those days medicine, like other arts and crafts, was primarily an itinerant vocation. The doctor came to a town, knocked at doors offering his services, and if there were enough sick people either he rented a shop somewhere on the market place and settled down for a while; or the townspeople, eager to hold him for a time, put a shop at his disposal. Patients came or were brought. Relatives and friends crowded the place watching the doctor as he examined and treated the sick. There must have been little privacy in the relationship between physician and patient, and we must imagine conditions very much as they still are in the Orient today. In some cases, of course, particularly when the patient was a rich man, the physician went to his residence.

We have seen that physicians were not licensed in antiquity, so that anybody could claim to be a doctor and treat patients for fees. How, then, could society distinguish a competent physician from a quack? Some doctors were known to a town because they had been there before and had established a reputation for themselves, thus winning the confidence of the people. But others were new to the place. How could they prove that they were not impostors but well-trained, honest craftsmen? The Hippocratic treatise *Prognosticon* gives an answer. It begins with the statement:

I hold that it is an excellent thing for a physician to practice forecasting. For if he discover and declare unaided by the side of his patients the present, the past, and the future,

and fill in the gaps in the account given by the sick, he will
be the more believed to understand the cases, so that men
will confidently entrust themselves to him for treatment.[2]

In other words, a physician seeing a patient was expected to be able to tell immediately what had happened to him, what his condition was, and what fate
had in store for him. If he could do this and if events
proved that he was correct, his reputation was established. Prognosis, prediction of the future course of a
disease, is what impresses the people most. This they
can check. The peculiar conditions of medical practice in the fifth century B.C. explain to a large extent
why the art of making prognoses was so highly developed in Hippocratic medicine.[3]

There must have been a great deal of competition
between physicians, as there was between other craftsmen. We hear that some doctors endeavored to impress
the people by dressing extravagantly and scenting
themselves. Others displayed spectacular instruments.
The Hippocratic writings condemn such practices
but the fact that they are mentioned proves that they
existed.

The Hippocratic physician was paid for his services, and since Greek society despised people who
worked for money his social position was not very
high. Yet among all the craftsmen he was held in the

2. *Prognostic* I; Loeb Classical Series. Hippocrates, II, 7.
3. Ludwig Edelstein in his book, *Peri Aeron und die Sammlung
der hippokratischen Schriften* (Berlin, 1931), has made a careful
study of medical practice in Hippocratic times and has drawn
our attention to all these facts.

highest esteem because health was considered one of the greatest goods.

In the early days of ancient Rome physicians were mostly slaves.[4] The big landowners had slaves who were skilled in definite crafts and those who knew how to treat disease brought a good price on the market, as much as a eunuch. Their medical knowledge was very primitive and treatment consisted mostly in the application of house remedies. When Greek physicians began to immigrate into Rome in the third century B.C. their superior knowledge soon became apparent, although many of them were adventurers and quacks. The Roman armies needed physicians and surgeons and efforts were made to attract Greek doctors. Julius Caesar, in 46 B.C., presented all freeborn Greek physicians on Roman soil with Roman citizenship, a great gift in a world in which foreigners had no rights of any kind. Augustus knighted his body-physician Musa. More privileges were extended to medical men. They were tax exempt, free of the duty of serving in the army, of the duty of boarding and lodging soldiers, and excused from assuming honorary offices. But since there was no state control of the practice of medicine, anybody could claim the privileges by calling himself a doctor. And so restrictions had to be made. Under Antoninus Pius a regulation was passed providing that only five, seven, or ten physicians, according to the size of the city, should be granted the privileges, and that they must present

4. Th. Meyer-Steineg, *Geschichte des römischen Aerztestandes* (Kiel, 1907).

their credentials to the authorities to obtain them. Such petitions are preserved in papyri from Egypt.[5]

This was the beginning of a state control of medicine in the Western World. The privileged physicians whose competence was certified by the authorities were the *valde docti*. In the second century A.D. the government helped physicians still more by providing rooms for them, and in the third century the state began to feel responsible for the training of physicians and appointed professors of medicine in Rome. In the sixth century there was a flourishing medical school in Ravenna, a Western Latin counterpart to Greek Alexandria.

The Hippocratic physician was a craftsman who sold his services to whoever was able to purchase them. In imperial Rome many physicians had salaried positions, at court, in the army, in gladiatorial schools, theaters, thermae, gardens, or were attached to a few families who paid them an annual stipend. Most doctors, however, were in private practice, where competition was fierce and unscrupulous. There were specialists for every organ and every treatment, and in the capital there were some who charged from $2,000 to $10,000 for special cures or operations.

In the Middle Ages conditions of medical practice changed radically. The surgeon who worked with his hands remained a craftsman and learned his art from a master, frequently his father. But as a rule physicians were clerics in the early Middle Ages, and the church provided a living for them so that they could

5. *Select Papyri* (1934), II, 270 ff. Loeb Classical Series.

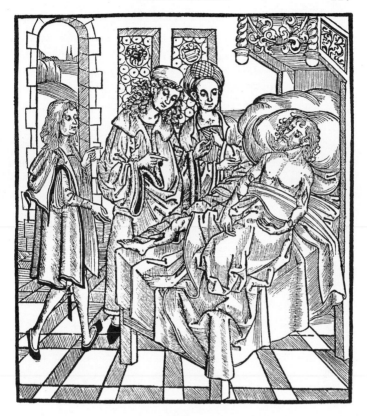

Fig. 16.

The Medieval Physician.

From Hieronymus Brunschwig, *Buch der Cirurgia,* 1497.

practice medicine as a charitable service. If gifts were offered, they were allowed to accept them, but they were not supposed to ask for them.[6]

6. E. Hirschfeld, "Deontologische Texte des frühen Mittelalters," *Archiv für Geschichte der Medizin,* XX (1928), 353–371.

Throughout the Middle Ages many physicians, because of their clerical status, were removed from economic considerations. But from the eleventh century
on laymen entered the profession in increasing numbers and this created a new situation. They were not
supported by the church and had to make a living.
This they did as a rule either by seeking a salaried
position as body-physician to some nobleman, lay or
ecclesiastical, or by entering the service of a city as
municipal doctor. And when they treated private patients they had to follow rigid codes, for in the mean-
time universities had been established and their medical faculties had full control of the practice of medicine.

The Western university developed from three different roots, from the municipal, the cathedral, and
the cloister school. A free association of teachers and
students grouped around the cathedral school of Paris
became the nucleus of that great university. A group
of lawyers and their students was the starting point
of the University of Bologna, and physicians teaching medicine established the universities of Salerno
and Montpellier. The origins were different, but the
end product was the same. When the medieval university was at its height in the early thirteenth century,
it owned no property. It had a charter and privileges
and enjoyed the protection of the church, but owned
no buildings and no endowments. It was free to shape
its own destiny and at liberty to move wherever conditions seemed most favorable.[7]

7. See Stephen d'Irsay, *Histoire des Universités* (Paris, 1933), I.

The medical faculty of the university trained physicians and controlled their actions, thus gradually assuming the same functions as the medieval craftsmen's guilds. Like the guild the faculty considered its task to be the transmission of a definite body of knowledge and skills, the preservation of pure traditions, the guarantee of high standards of quality, and the elimination of competition by strictly regulating prices.

The medieval world was a static world. Created by God in a definite order for all times to come, it was the best possible world. Man was born with a divine mission to fulfil. Salvation, not the accumulation of wealth, was his purpose. It was an authoritarian world dominated in all its aspects by the church. Professions were vocations implying duties toward God and fellowmen. Adjustments had to be made because members of the professions had to live, and food and industrial products had to be paid for in money. But stipends and salaries provided, as a rule, the means of subsistence. And when a physician had to charge a fee it was done according to strict and binding tariffs.

Abuses occurred, in medicine as everywhere, and history knows of greedy physicians, surgeons, and pharmacists. They were exceptions and their actions were strongly condemned by a society in which money did not give prestige.

Again conditions changed radically about the sixteenth century, when there arose a new economic order, appealing to the individualist in man and calling for free initiative, free trade, free competition. Such

an order could not develop under the rigid regulations of the medieval world. Traditional authorities
were opposed and the most powerful among them, the
church, was "reformed." A new political philosophy
was born, the philosophy of liberalism. The craftsmen's guilds lost their political and economic power
while retaining their welfare institutions. But the
universities for a long time refused to adapt themselves to the new conditions, persistently clinging to
medieval forms and traditions. This hastened the
foundation of academies which were to become the
centers of scientific research. Medical faculties gradually lost their power to control the practice of medicine, which in many countries was taken over by the
state. State medical boards were founded. They licensed physicians to practice and became the advisers
of government in matters of health. A new science,
established and cultivated by a rapidly growing
middle class, was soon to revolutionize not only medicine but also the entire field of technology.

The physician found himself at the mercy of a
competitive world which was utterly strange to him.
Professions were no longer considered divine missions
but simply means of making a living. Once more, as
had been the case in antiquity, the doctor had to sell
his services on the open market. But now the situation was totally different. In antiquity the physician
sold his services to whoever could pay for them and
nobody cared about the indigent sick. Now, however,
after many centuries of Christianity, the idea was
generally accepted that everybody, whether rich or

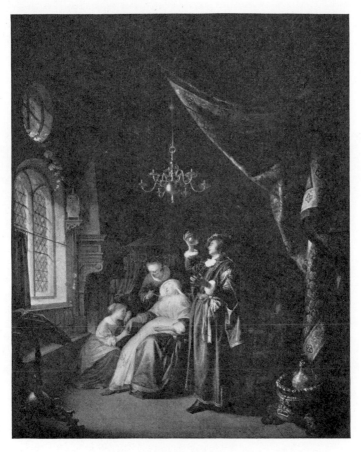

Fig. 17.

The Physician in the Seventeenth Century.

Painting by Gerard Douw.

poor, should have all the medical services he needed. Yet only a very few people could afford to purchase medical care, and charitable institutions although increased could not possibly solve the problem.

The inherent contradictions of such a system became all too apparent. It was soon realized that medical services could not be valued solely in terms of money. An hour's conversation may save a patient's life, while a major operation may be wasted. For a long time physicians refused to accept the challenge of the new economic order and strenuously resisted developments. As heretofore they sought salaried positions as body-physicians or in government services, in order to be independent and free to serve the poor or to devote part of their activities to research and similar occupations. With the rise of the middle class, physicians endeavored to attach themselves to a number of such families. The family doctor is the democratic form of the body-physician. In European countries until the end of the nineteenth century many family doctors never wrote a bill. Families sent to their doctor, around Christmas time, what they could afford or considered fair, and this was enough to secure him a modest but decent living and to allow him to treat indigent patients without remuneration.

The physicians' attempt to preserve medieval ideals of service in a world ruled by iron economic necessities was heroic but was doomed to failure. The situation became still more complicated during the nineteenth and twentieth centuries when, as a result of industrialization, the needy population increased tre-

mendously and at the same time the cost of medical
care was rising, largely because of the progress of
medical science. Against his will and in spite of des-
perate resistance the physician found himself in a

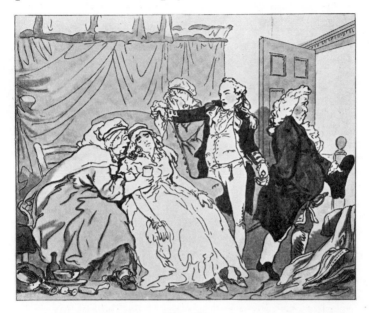

Fig. 18.

The Dying Patient or the Doctor's Last Fee.

By J. Rowlandson, 1786.

harshly competitive business. When this was generally realized, although it was not openly admitted,
medical societies were organized, and codes of ethics
and etiquette were promulgated to safeguard the
profession against some of the worst features of com-

petition, such as advertising, underbidding, fee-split-ting, taking patients away from a colleague, and similar procedures. Physicians still looked back to medieval ideals, still were willing to attend indigent patients free of charge, but an untenable situation arose. Unless special adjustments were made, either large sections of the population would remain unat-tended or the medical profession must be ruined.

At this point we must consider another line of de-velopment. Medicine originally was a private rela-tionship between physician and patient. What hap-pened between the two did not concern anybody else. But both physician and patient were members of a society and for a long time the tendency has been for medicine to become a social institution. Society has always been interested in the physician's behavior for the simple reason that the practice of medicine gives the physician tremendous power over man. The phy-sician knows poisons; biological, physical, and chemi-cal forces of high potency are placed freely in his hands, and he enters many houses, where secrets are divulged to him that the patient would not reveal to anybody else. This all gives him a unique power over people, a power whose misuse would quite evidently be a serious menace to society. Therefore, society has at all times tried to protect itself against such misuse. In ancient Babylonia, around 2000 B.C., the Code of Hammurabi declared the physician, or rather the surgeon, liable for his acts.[8] If his operation suc-

8. Chilperic Edwards, *The Hammurabi Code* (London, 1921), p. 40.

ceeded he was remunerated according to a tariff, the fee being determined by the social status of the patient. If it failed, however, he was punished, and this was done again according to the social status of the patient. If the victim was a free man, the surgeon was prevented from further operating once and for all: his right hand was cut off. If the victim was a slave he was to be replaced by another slave.

In no profession is ignorance so dangerous as in the medical profession. A wrong legal judgment may be corrected by a higher court. A wrong diagnosis or treatment may result in the patient's death. Little wonder that society tried to protect itself against ignorant physicians by setting definite standards which must be met before a man could call himself a physician and practice medicine.[9] The idea of licensing physicians took root in the Middle Ages, but its origin can be traced back to antiquity. The Avesta, the sacred book of the Persians, contains a very significant passage:

36 (94) Maker of the material world, thou Holy One! If a worshipper of Mazda want to practice the art of healing, on whom shall he first prove his skill?—on worshippers of Mazda or on worshippers of the Daêvas?—

37 (96) Ahura Mazda answered: "On worshippers of the Daêvas shall he first prove himself, rather than on worshippers of Mazda. If he treat with the knife a worshipper of the Daêvas and he die; if he treat with the knife a second worshipper of the Daêvas and he die; if he treat with the knife for the third time a worshipper of the Daêvas and he

9. H. E. Sigerist, "The History of Medical Licensure," *Journal of the American Medical Association*, CIV (1935), 1057–1060.

die, he is unfit to practice the art of healing forever and
ever.

38 (99) "Let him therefore never attend any worshipper
of Mazda; let him never treat with the knife any worshipper of Mazda, nor wound him with the knife. If he shall
ever attend any worshipper of Mazda, if he shall ever treat
with the knife any worshipper of Mazda and wound him
with the knife, he shall pay for it the same penalty as is
paid for wilful murder.

39 (102) "If he treat with the knife a worshipper of the
Daêvas and he recover; if he treat with the knife the second
worshipper of the Daêvas and he recover; if for the third
time he treat with the knife a worshipper of the Daêvas and
he recover; then he is fit to practice the art of healing forever and ever.

40 (104) "He may henceforth at his will attend worshippers of Mazda; he may at his will treat with the knife
worshippers of Mazda, and heal them with the knife."[10]

We have already mentioned the privileges extended
to a limited number of qualified Roman physicians.
In the Arabic world in 931 A.D. the Caliph Al-
Muqtadir decided that no one should practice medicine in the capital, in Bagdad, unless he had been examined by the physician Sinan ibn Thabit of Har-
ran. A few generally respected physicians were ex-
empted from these examinations, but all the others—
and it is said that there were more than eight hundred
and sixty physicians in Bagdad at the time—had to
submit themselves to the test. It is not known whether
this attempt was repeated by the later caliphs.[11]

10. "The Zend Avesta," I. *The Vendidad,* J. Darmesteter, ed., in
"Sacred Books of the East," F. M. Müller, ed. (Oxford, 1880), IV,
83–84.

11. E. G. Browne, *Arabian Medicine* (New York, 1921), p. 40.

Medical licensure became a permanent institution in the West beginning with the Middle Ages and its history is intimately connected with the rise of the university. The first regulations were issued in connection with the first medical faculty of the Western World, the School of Salerno. In 1140 the Norman king Roger issued an order stating:

Who, from now on, wishes to practice medicine, has to present himself before our officials and examiners, in order to pass their judgment. Should he be bold enough to disregard this, he will be punished by imprisonment and confiscation of his entire property. In this way we are taking care that our subjects are not endangered by the inexperience of the physicians.

Nobody dare practice medicine unless he has been found fit by the convention of the Salernitan masters.

From 1231 to 1240 the Hohenstaufen emperor Frederick II published his *Constitutiones Imperiales*, a code based on the old Norman codes but adding new laws. The regulations concerning physicians are very detailed, prescribing a curriculum of three years of logic and five years of medicine, supplemented by a practical year. After these nine years of study the candidate was examined by the Salernitan masters in the presence of representatives of the state. Heavy penalties threatened whoever practiced without a license. Other universities followed Salerno's example, and when medical faculties lost their powers state boards assumed the task of protecting society against the ignorance and inexperience of physicians.

Society had still other means for protecting itself

against abuse of the physician's power. In most countries the penal code protects germinating life, guards the patient's secrets, requires the consent of the patient for being operated on, and makes the physician liable for damage due to negligence.[12]

Society, however, did not limit itself to protective measures against medical abuses. It took active steps to enforce health through administrative procedures. The physician was called upon to act as the medical expert in creating conditions for health. He thus became an administrator who protected society against disease by improving sanitary conditions, establishing quarantines and similar measures. As we have already seen, public health services in the course of time assumed more and more medical tasks, being obliged to step in wherever private competitive medicine was unable to solve a problem. Since under the new system private practitioners had to be paid for every single service, and because many, and particularly chronic, patients could not possibly do so, public services were expected also to assume responsibility for most tubercular, mental, and many other chronic patients. In such services the public physician was not only an administrator but a therapeutist as well. Every civilized country, including the United States, today undertakes a large and steadily increasing amount of state medicine and public medical services, financed through taxation, and it is these which are largely responsible for improved health conditions.

12. L. Ebermayer, "Der Arzt in Gesetz und Rechtsgebung," in *Der Arzt und der Staat,* "Vorträge des Instituts für Geschichte der Medizin an der Universität Leipzig" (Leipzig, 1929), II, 45–59.

While medical science progressed, the scope of medicine broadened considerably. Much of the administration of justice is impossible without the cooperation of the physician, who is the scientific adviser to the court. He must ascertain the cause of a man's death and the circumstances under which death occurred. If a corpse is found in a pond, it is the physician's task to determine whether the man was drowned in the pond or whether he was thrown into it as a cadaver, and in addition he must be able to tell how long the corpse has been in the water. The court's action depends entirely on the physician's expert advice. This is the wide field of forensic medicine, which has developed tremendously in recent years and has contributed a great deal to legal security.

The physician is also psychological adviser to the court. Aided by the growing psychological and psychopathological knowledge, the sense of justice has evolved and today the view is generally held that a man cannot be made responsible for an offense committed while his mind worked abnormally as a result of illness. It is the psychiatrist's task to determine the degree of responsibility of an offender, and again the court's action may be influenced by the physician's findings.

Recent developments in jurisprudence have created a still greater demand for psychiatric advice. In former centuries society by sentencing a criminal took vengeance on him and punished him for his action. Today the judge in passing sentence intends to protect society and to rehabilitate the offender. He tries

to readjust him to his social environment so that he
may again become a useful member of society. Physician and judge act with somewhat the same intention.
The patient and the criminal offender are, in different ways, a burden on society: each has become useless and may even be dangerous, both must be rehabili-
tated in society's and in their own interest. Since the
causes are different, the methods of treatment must
differ: but the goal is the same for physician and
judge.

If the judge wishes to pass a sentence that will
serve its purpose, he ought to know the offender intimately and on the basis of a detailed social, psychological, and in many instances also a physical case
history. He should know the etiology of the case under treatment, and this would necessitate the coöperation of a physician, whose help would also be required
in determining the kind and measure of the sentence.
The same sentence passed for the same offense may
have opposite results on different individuals. The
psychiatrist's coöperation is particularly fruitful in
juvenile courts because the reëducation of young individuals is easier than that of adults.

I mentioned in a previous chapter that the physician is playing an increasingly important part in
education. He is not only responsible for the physical
development of children but for their mental adjustments as well. Mental hygiene is one of the most
promising fields of medicine and education.

The scope of medicine also broadened considerably
as a result of economic developments. Before the in-

dustrial revolution the structure of social life was relatively simple. A farm or a craftsman's household was a more or less self-contained unit. Cities were generally small, the rhythm of life was slow, and the individual moved in a narrowly limited sphere. The development of industry radically changed all this. Society became highly differentiated and specialized. Today we no longer store food over the winter because we can buy it fresh or preserved within easy reach of our homes. Water, light, and heat are brought to the house and we need not bother about the disposal of refuse and sewage. We have created agencies to do the work for us. This means, however, that in a modern community everybody depends on everybody else. A general strike paralyzes a city within twenty-four hours.

Work is an essential factor of health. It balances and gives significance to our lives, ennobling them and permitting man to create those material and cultural values without which human existence would be meaningless. It is good that man must work in order to live. But work can also be harmful, and the development of industry created a vast array of new hazards that threatened not only the worker's health and life but also that of society at large. Industry has brought man very close to physical and chemical forces of tremendous potency. It has become the physician's duty to protect him against these new hazards and the task is one of such magnitude that the co-operation of scientists and engineers is required. The protection of labor, the creation of sound working conditions, of a clean and healthy factory atmosphere, is one of the primary tasks of medicine today. Every factory should have physicians on its staff but in the

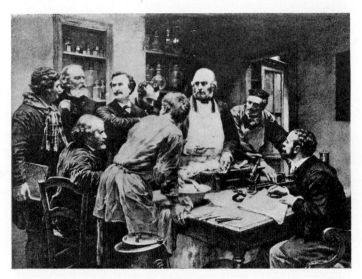

Fig. 19.

The Physician and Scientist.

Claude Bernard's laboratory.

From the painting by Léon Lhermitte.

United States, one of the most highly industrialized countries in the world, the majority of industrial enterprises have no medical facilities of any kind.[13]

Every new industry has brought with it new health problems, and since industry is constantly developing

13. *Report of the Technical Committee on Medical Care* (Washington, 1938).

the physician is compelled to face new problems every day. And while they all concern the people's health and welfare, their solution is by no means exclusively medical. In spite of all safety devices, some industries will remain harmful to health. The solution of such problems obviously lies in the reduction of working hours to six, five, or possibly even four hours a day without reduction of wages, in the granting of vacations on full pay, and in the provision of means for rest and recreation. These are not strictly medical problems but problems of labor policy. The physician, however, who is familiar with conditions and knows the evil effects of such work on the people's health must assume leadership in the struggle for the improvement of conditions. His concern is not whether an enterprise is profitable or not. His place is with the workers, whose protector he is.

Industry has affected the people's health not only directly through the process of production but also indirectly by creating certain living conditions. We have mentioned how wretched these conditions were in the beginning of industrialization and what a serious health problem they constituted. Since then they have been improved in some cases, but by no means everywhere, and they are far from being stable at a high level. Flourishing industrial communities have been wiped out by economic depressions.[14] I have seen cities in the United States that remind one of Pompeii and Herculaneum, but the volcano that destroyed them

14. See Eileen Wilkinson's stirring book, *The Town That Was Murdered: The Life-Story of Jarrow* (London, 1939).

was man-made and its eruption might have been prevented by social planning. High as a worker's standard of living may be at certain times, he is never secure. The next crisis wipes out his savings, destroys his standard, and exposes him to the physical and mental agony of unemployment. Eager to work and to provide a decent living for his family, he becomes useless, undesirable, perhaps a recipient of charity for many years, and this, as has been pointed out countless times, in a world that has food for everybody, raw materials and factories, hands and brains able to produce all the commodities that people could possibly desire. If he is still able to think, he will curse a system that deprives him of his elementary right to work.

Does that concern the physician? Of course it does. The social causes of illness are just as important as the physical ones. Etiological therapy means more than killing a few bugs. The medical officer of health and the practitioners of a distressed area are the natural advocates of the people. They well know the factors that paralyze all their efforts. They are not only scientists but also responsible citizens, and if they did not raise their voice, who else should?

Science has progressed and technology has developed. Industry has adopted methods of mass production, involving division of labor and such innovations as the conveyer-belt system. Enormous quantities of raw materials are needed to feed the machine, and new foreign markets to absorb the products. The result is imperialism and wars; wars fought scientifically, with cannon, airplanes, and tanks produced on conveyers by industry, according to the last methods of technology, themselves based on the most recent progress of science. Millions of people are killed, other millions die of starvation and pestilence.

Does that concern the physician? The World War of 1914–18 destroyed almost as many human lives as the epidemic of influenza. And like influenza, it selected not weaklings but strong individuals in the prime of life. War is a social disease, like poverty or crime. When it breaks out it reminds us that we are still in the initial stages, in the prehistory of civilization, not far removed from savagery. It reminds us that although we like to play with science and kill with scientific weapons, we have not yet learned to approach the basic problems of social life—production, distribution, and consumption—scientifically. If a physician believes in his work he cannot but abhor war, which is the negation of all his efforts. When war comes he of course will do his best to alleviate the sufferings that stupidity, inefficiency, and greed have brought upon his fellowmen. And he is fortunate in that he himself is not obliged to kill. We whose lifetime falls into a period of transition, when a decaying world is committing deliberate suicide, have all spent years in uniform or shall do so. But the physician has still another task, namely, to side passionately with life against death, to fight the obvious causes of war and to help in paving the way for a better world. And he should remember that open war, after all, is merely the acute form of a disease which in its chronic form is endemic in our society. Even in the most peaceful years thousands of human beings are oppressed, crushed, and starved out in a war that is not so spec-

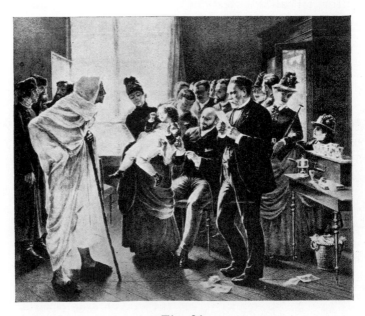

Fig. 20.

Immunization Clinic.

Immunization against rabies in Pasteur's laboratory.

From the painting by Laurent Grell.

tacular as the formal one but just as deadly. There is a front for the physician here, too.

Industrial work is wage work and under finance capitalism the men at the head of an enterprise are not the owners of the plant but the salaried employees of stockholders. The result is that today in highly industrialized countries like the United States, four fifths of all gainfully employed persons are wage earners or salaried employees. In other words: eighty per cent of all breadwinners depend for an income on the labor market. They have a job today but may lose it tomorrow. And we know how many people have actually lost their jobs in recent years.

This is a totally new situation. The structure of our present society is basically different from what it was before the industrial era when only one out of five gainfully employed persons was a wage earner and four owned their means of production and were independent farmers, artisans, or business people.

It is fairly obvious that the present situation creates a strong feeling of insecurity and as a result an equally strong demand for social security. The wage earner is perfectly willing to pay according to his ability for whatever services he gets, including medical care, but he must have a system that permits him to meet costs through some kind of periodic payments. And he must through his payments acquire a right to these services and the certainty that he will not be deprived of them when conditions of the labor market deny him the chance to work. He does not want charity. What he wants is the right to work, to perform work that will permit him to satisfy his and his family's basic needs. A society that is unable to provide socially useful work to all its members rests on a shaky foundation and is bound sooner or later to collapse. I think the events of the last ten years have demonstrated this unmistakably.

As a result of all these developments the physician finds himself in a precarious situation. In the last seventy years medical science has advanced more than ever before in history. In order to acquire the prescribed minimum of knowledge and skills the student must spend almost ten years on studies in college, medical school, and hospital, and must invest a considerable capital in order to become a doctor. When at last he is qualified to practice, he must sell his services on the open market to a society that consists mostly of wage earners who have no security of income. He is not free to choose the place in which he wishes to practice. He cannot settle down where his services are needed most urgently, but must select a community that is able to support him and to provide for him the standard of living to which he feels himself entitled after so many years of study and such great sacrifices. We know that the distribution of physicians is not determined by need but by the per capita spendable income of the population. Even when he has selected the economically right kind of community the young doctor is often unable to apply all he has learned in medical school. Necessary examinations and treatments must be omitted because the equipment is unavailable or because they are too costly to the patient. Many physicians try to solve their problem by investing more money in studies and spending a few more years in hospitals. They become specialists and this entitles them to higher fees. But in order to obtain them they must practice in the larger cities, with the result that there are more specialists than are needed and they are badly distributed.

Under such a system large sections of the population have no medical care at all or certainly not enough. The technology of medicine has outrun its sociology. Many health problems have been solved medically but remain socially untouched, thus defeating the progress and wasting the gains of medical science.

There is only one solution to the problem. We are convinced that the people's health is important and that it is a senseless waste of human happiness and wealth to have thousands of people needlessly sick and thousands dying prematurely. We no longer accept the Greek view that health is a privilege of the rich, but agree with the medieval idea that everybody, rich and poor, should have all the medical care that science can give. There is only one way of achieving this: the physician must be removed from the sphere of competitive business. He must be liberated from the economic bonds that were forced upon him by a system which is incompatible with the character of medical service as we conceive it today. We cannot think of a minister of the church, a judge, or a professor selling his services on the open market. The physician is doing work of great social significance and must be guaranteed in exchange complete social security and the standard of living to which his education entitles him. He must be free from economic worries so that he can devote all his energy, intelligence, and skill to his great task. It is not by accident that most progress in medicine has been achieved by physicians in salaried positions.

Private competitive medicine cannot satisfy the health needs of a nation. This was recognized long ago, and this is why public health services were established in every country and developed more rapidly as the nation became more conscious of health. This is why charity services had to be maintained although charity is a poor principle of organization because it may fail in times of economic stress when help is most urgently needed. This is why special regulations had to be made to protect the worker and to guarantee him medical aid and compensation when he is the victim of industrial accidents and occupational diseases. But even so, private competitive medicine is left in charge of most of the nation's health work, is responsible for it, and is facing a task which it is unable to solve.

The problem is world-wide and long ago attempts were made in many countries to organize the services of the practitioner and to "decommercialize" them. The idea was to guarantee medical care to every wage earner, and to every practitioner adequate remuneration for his work. The method consisted in spreading the risks among as many people as possible and pooling the resources of large groups. As we have seen, Germany in 1883 was the first country to introduce compulsory sickness insurance. The example was followed by almost all European and by a number of American countries. This is not the place to discuss and criticize the various insurance systems,[15] but it is fair to state that sickness insurance brought doctors to many thousands of people who had never had them before and that it increased the physicians' incomes considerably.

Most present insurance systems have serious defects which are due to a simple cause. They are too conservative. They were established with the idea of financing the extension of existing services to groups which did not have them before. People failed to realize that the application of a new medical science to a new type of society required new forms of service. The result was that in many countries insurance did not improve health services but merely extended them in their traditional haphazard form.

Another much more radical attempt to organize the physicians' services can be traced back to 1818. In that year the German duchy of Nassau established a complete system of public medicine by appointing physicians as civil servants.[16] Each one of the twenty-eight districts had a physician in chief (*Medizinal-rat*) with two assistant physicians and one or two assistant surgeons. Their salaries were raised through a special tax. This made medical care available to all. The system was in operation until 1861, when Nassau lost its independence and became a province of Prus-

15. I shall do it in a book on *Medical Economics,* a series of lectures delivered at the University of the Witwatersrand in Johannesburg, South Africa.

16. See Kurt Finkenrath, *Sozialismus im Heilwesen: Eine geschichtliche Betrachtung des Medizinalwesens im Herzogtum Nassau von 1800–1866* (Berlin, 1930).

sia. When it was abandoned endless petitions were sent to Berlin by the people of Nassau requesting the authorities to let them retain their system of medical care, but the Prussian government insisted on uniformity in administrative matters.

Three years later, in 1864, medical care was made a public service in the rural districts of Russia. The administration of welfare, public health, and education was turned over to the zemstvos, the local district assemblies. Hospitals and medical stations were owned and operated by the zemstvo. Physicians and other medical personnel were government officials in the service of the zemstvo. Taxation provided the funds. Physicians were paid salaries, very often had free living quarters, were paid traveling expenses and entitled to a pension when they retired.

There were splendid characters among these zemstvo doctors. The businessman type of physician obviously remained in the city, but many young people, men and women, went to the country with great enthusiasm to serve their fellowmen. Chekhov, who was a zemstvo physician himself, has pictured them in many novels and plays.

Zemstvo medicine was the foundation upon which the Soviet Union erected its system of medicine.[17] It is a system under which the protection of the people's health has become a public service in all its aspects. All health services are free and therefore available to everybody. All health activities are directed by cen-

17. H. E. Sigerist, *Socialized Medicine in the Soviet Union* (New York, 1937).

tral agencies which not only determine policies but also train the personnel they need and produce its technical equipment. Medical services are organized around health centers which are responsible for the people they are called to protect and endeavor to prevent illness wherever this can be done. Health work is carried out according to definite plans and with the broad participation of the people.

History points out the direction in which medicine is moving. The physician's knowledge is no longer based on theology or philosophy but on science. Scientific research will therefore remain the rich source that supplies the physician with ever-improved views, methods, and techniques for the protection of health and the fight against disease. Research must be promoted by all means available. But scientific knowledge alone is not enough. Physician and patient do not meet on a lone island but are both members of a highly differentiated society. Hence scientific research must be supplemented by sociological research which studies the life cycle of man in his social environment and investigates factors favorable or detrimental to health and methods of social readjustment.

Medicine already is sufficiently advanced to give the physician the means necessary for the practice of preventive medicine on a large scale. Prevention of disease must become the goal of every physician whatever his status may be. The barriers between preventive and curative medicine must be broken down.

The general practitioner will remain the core of the medical profession, but alone, left to himself, he is

lost and cannot possibly practice scientific medicine.
He needs the backing of a health center or hospital
and a group of specialists whose help and advice he
can seek. Practice tomorrow will of necessity be group
practice, organized around a health center which will
have health stations as outposts in strategic points of
the district. The people need more than a family doctor; they need a family health center where physicians
will not wait until a sick man calls on them but from
where they will go out into the homes and working
places in order to help the people before illness strikes.
No longer will the doctor be economically dependent
on his patients, forced to exploit their illness and suffering. Whether such a health center should be financed through taxation or compulsory or voluntary
insurance is a secondary consideration which will depend on circumstances.

I am convinced that medicine, like education, will
ultimately become a public service in every civilized
country. All trends are in that direction. Under such
a system medicine can fully apply all scientific means
at its disposal and can reach the entire population.
Under it, moreover, the risks are spread among the
largest possible number of people and their resources
are pooled.

At what time such a point will be reached in the
various countries will depend on economic, social, and
political developments. It may be sooner than we
commonly expect. The war which broke out in 1939
will destroy the *laissez faire* attitude once and for all

and will force social adjustments that have been neglected in the past.

The scope of medicine has indeed broadened. There is today hardly a field of human endeavor that does not require the physician's advice at some time or other. No longer a shaman, priest, craftsman, or cleric, he must be more than a mere scientist. We begin to perceive the outline of a new physician. Scientist and social worker, prepared to coöperate in teamwork and in close touch with the people he serves; a friend and leader, he will direct all his efforts toward the prevention of disease and become a therapist when prevention has broken down—the social physician protecting the people and guiding them to a healthier and happier life.

INDEX OF NAMES